Super Easy
AYURVEDIC CLEANSING

A Beginner's Guide to Ayurveda for Natural Healing and Balance

....
KIMBERLY LARSON
....

NEW SHOE PRESS

Brimming with creative inspiration, how-to projects, and useful information to enrich your everyday life, quarto.com is a favorite destination for those pursuing their interests and passions.

First Published in 2022 by New Shoe Press, an imprint of The Quarto Group, 100 Cummings Center, Suite 265-D, Beverly, MA 01915, USA.
T (978) 282-9590 F (978) 283-2742 **Quarto.com**

New Shoe Press titles are also available at discount for retail, wholesale, promotional, and bulk purchase. For details, contact the Special Sales Manager by email at specialsales@ quarto.com or by mail at The Quarto Group, Attn: Special Sales Manager, 100 Cummings Center, Suite 265-D, Beverly, MA 01915, USA.

ISBN: 978-0-7603-8011-6
eISBN: 978-0-7603-8012-3

The content in this book was previously published in *The Simple, Healing Cleanse* (Fair Winds Press 2016) by Kimberly Larson.

Library of Congress Cataloging-in-Publication Data available.

Photography: Michelle Allen Photography//www.michellempls.com

The information in this book is for educational purposes only. It is not intended to replace the advice of a physician or medical practitioner. Please see your health-care provider before beginning any new health program.

Contents

Foreword 4

Introduction 6

PART I
FUNDAMENTALS OF HEALTH
& BALANCE 9

Chapter One
The Essence of Ayurveda 11

Chapter Two
Understanding Your Body-Mind Type 17

Chapter Three
Foods for Balance 29

Chapter Four
Why Do We Need to Cleanse? 41

PART II
CLEANSING FOR YOUR
BODY-MIND TYPE 51

Chapter Five
Simple Eating for Everyone 53

Chapter Six
Grounding Cleanse & Diet 69

Chapter Seven
Lightening Cleanse & Diet 95

Chapter Eight
Cooling Cleanse & Diet 116

Chapter Nine
Taking It Deeper:
Traditional Ayurvedic Cleansing 133

Appendix 138

Index 142

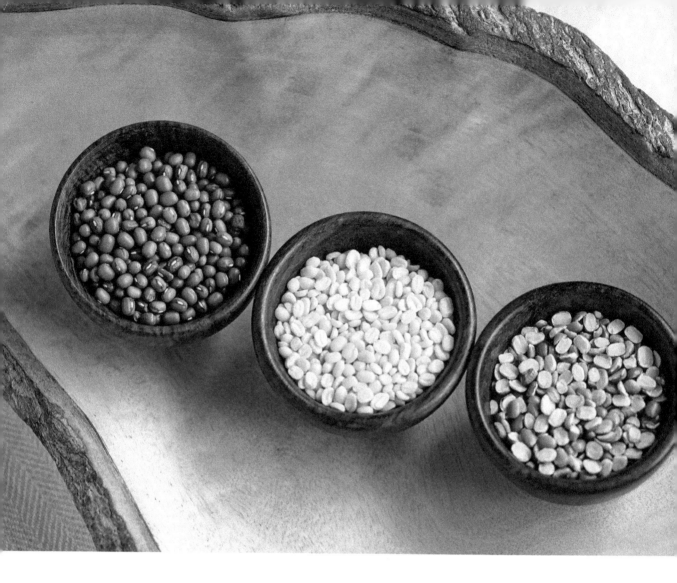

Foreword

Public health is the science and art of supporting the health and quality of life in a community. Though methods vary greatly among cultures, in general, public health practices aim to reach community members in a meaningful way—so that we as individuals change our behavior for the better. When we change, our communities change. When our communities change, our countries change. When our countries change, our world changes. Big change, as we so often hear, does indeed begin with each one of us. One of the most creative ways to reach individuals through public health is one I came across when I first studied health in India in 1988.

In India, if you are a very observant Hindu, you celebrate more religious holidays than there are days in a year. Every single day has particular significance according to its position in the lunar calendar. Celebrations of each day range from modest affairs with minimal rituals to elaborate celebrations in which millions of people participate. An individual's reason to celebrate might be to nourish one's relationship to spiritual practices, to maintain religious protocol, or simply to not irritate family or community sensibilities. But there are also positive large, "public health" scale, side effects of each individual's participation. Why? Dietary restrictions or observances often accompany holidays—typically in the form of a fast. For example, during a one-day holiday, a celebrant is enjoined to fast until the evening—and then break the fast only with certain simple foods. Giving the digestive system a mini break in this way provides a small, gentle cleanse. In addition to these shorter fasts and festivals, some festivals are held during seasonal transitions and require more lengthy fasts. During the nine-day holiday of Navaratri, for example, celebrants fast on either liquids or only certain easily-digestible foods. This holiday occurs multiple times a year, but the autumn and spring Navaratris are the most widely observed.

Because the benefits of occasional fasting, especially during seasonal transitions, has been well known to Ayurveda in India for millennia, it is widely believed that the dietary and lifestyle observances that accompany holidays—especially ones that occur during seasonal transitions—were consciously instituted to support public health. If people fast or simplify their diet during the changes of season—times when disease is more apt to be initiated—it allows the body and mind to gently cleanse and better adapt to the rhythms and realities of the new season. Tying these measures to religious holidays helped ensure that the population—whether educated about good health practices or not—would be obliged to adopt them and therefore potentially

remain healthier. Although these practices may not be as strictly or widely practiced now, many Hindus still observe them. One recent example is that of India's Prime Minister Narendra Modi, who has, for decades, famously fasted on only liquids during Navaratri—even when it coincided with his maiden trip to the United States in the Fall of 2014, when he was sixty-four years old.

Though we in the West may not share the religion that initiated such fasts, we can still reap the benefits to mental, emotional, and spiritual health that these practices generate. Taking time to cleanse in a safe and gentle way, simplifying not only our diets but also fasting from the stimulation and demands of our daily responsibilities, allowing our attention to be stilled—or at least grow more still for a brief interlude—can refresh our energy, perspective, and relationship to life.

As individuals, we have the opportunity to educate ourselves about the wisdom of such practices and adopt them ourselves. This book can serve as a guide on how to calm and focus our attention, listen to and understand our bodies, simplify our diets, adopt gentle cleansing techniques, and internalize the value of doing so. Through these practices, our health can improve. Because our health also affects our families and our communities, we do change the world by changing ourselves.

So, happy holidays . . . whatever time of year you choose to celebrate good mental, spiritual, and physical health.

in love,
dr. claudia welch
doctor of oriental medicine

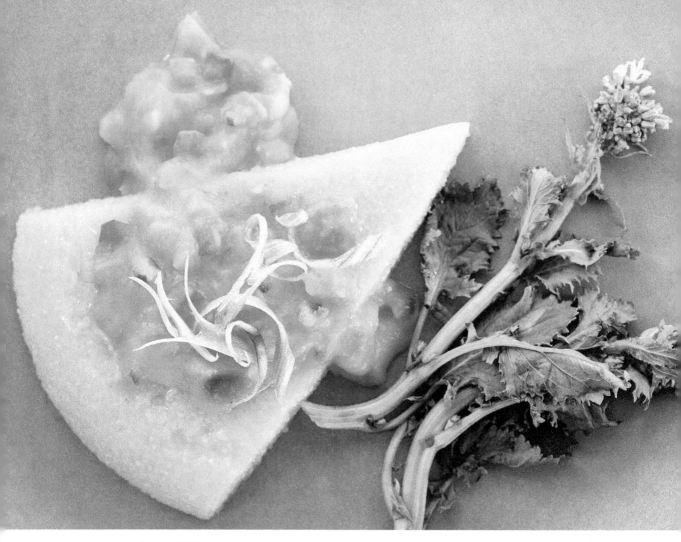

Lighten Up Polenta with Squash Sauce, page 112.

Introduction

Health is a state of being that includes our physical, mental, and emotional selves. We can have good health in which the body feels strong and vibrant, the mind is calm, and the emotions are stable and positive, or we can have poor health in which all components of our being show signs of imbalance. Making a choice about your personal state of being can feel overwhelming, because the amount of information about health, diet, and lifestyle choices available to anyone with technology-savvy fingertips can be mind-boggling and conflicting. Until I was introduced to the holistic system of medicine known as Ayurveda, I felt like I was randomly grasping at straws to choose which practices I should incorporate for my own health. But once I understood the intuitive, personalized Ayurvedic system, I could see that each diet, lifestyle, or cleanse out there is "healthy" for someone.

Cleansing is one practice that is often used to create better health—some people cleanse to lose weight, while others cleanse to improve the removal of byproducts from cellular metabolism, accumulations from poor diet, toxins in their food or environment, or qualities increased during each season of the year. However, this process intended to create better health can sometimes do the opposite.

I recall my first "cleanse," during which I drank only water for five days. A stranger told me how wonderful he felt after doing it, so I decided to try it. I did not have a framework to help me decide whether this would be a good idea for me; it definitely was not, and now, with knowledge of Ayurveda, I can see why. I was already thin and light in frame; it was a cooler than average autumn and I ended up chilled to the bone, ungrounded, and anxious from the lightening effects of the cleanse. This is an example of how practices meant to create better health can do the opposite if they are not chosen specifically for a person. The Ayurvedic framework can provide this personalized understanding.

After a decade as an Ayurvedic practitioner, I believe that people must address two factors before undertaking any cleanse. The first is to understand which diet will support health for you in your typical, everyday life and to use that knowledge to prepare food to nourish yourself. This baseline diet of personalized, healthful eating is important, because each one of us is different and therefore has different needs. We must meet those needs before we can prepare to undertake a cleanse. The second factor is to understand which type of cleanse is right for you, given your current state of health. The Ayurvedic principles explained in this book will provide the information needed to make knowledgeable decisions.

This book provides more than fifty recipes for personalized, healthful daily living as well as for times of cleansing. You can use the recipes for a seasonal everyday diet to maintain health by following the lightening recipes for spring, the cooling recipes for summer, and the grounding recipes for autumn. If you are feeling off or unhealthy, this book will help you determine your body type according to the Ayurvedic system and how your body may be out of balance. With that knowledge, you can create a daily diet to restore balance by choosing the modifications in each recipe that are appropriate for your body type. Part I of this book will give you the tools to understand your basic body-mind type and your current imbalance so that you can make good foundational choices about food.

You can also use these recipes when following the 31-day cleansing protocol, outlined in Part II. Designed to assist you in creating more awareness about food and relearning how to eat every day, the protocol will improve your lifelong health and help you to make conscious choices as you prepare to cleanse. It will then guide you through a gentle Ayurvedic cleanse and describe how to end the cleanse easily and safely. During this process, the recipes you choose can help right any imbalance you might have, so that your food becomes like medicine.

All of this knowledge is useless if someone cannot apply it. Knowing what food is good for you is the first step, but finding simple, easy recipes and time to prepare them is another. These recipes are from my personal collection, created to inspire many clients over the years to care for themselves by cooking. My cooking tips eliminate 90 percent of the effort and time in the kitchen—and that is the "magic" that makes vibrant health attainable for even the busiest bee. I hope that this book and the tradition of Ayurveda inspire good health for you and your family for years to come.

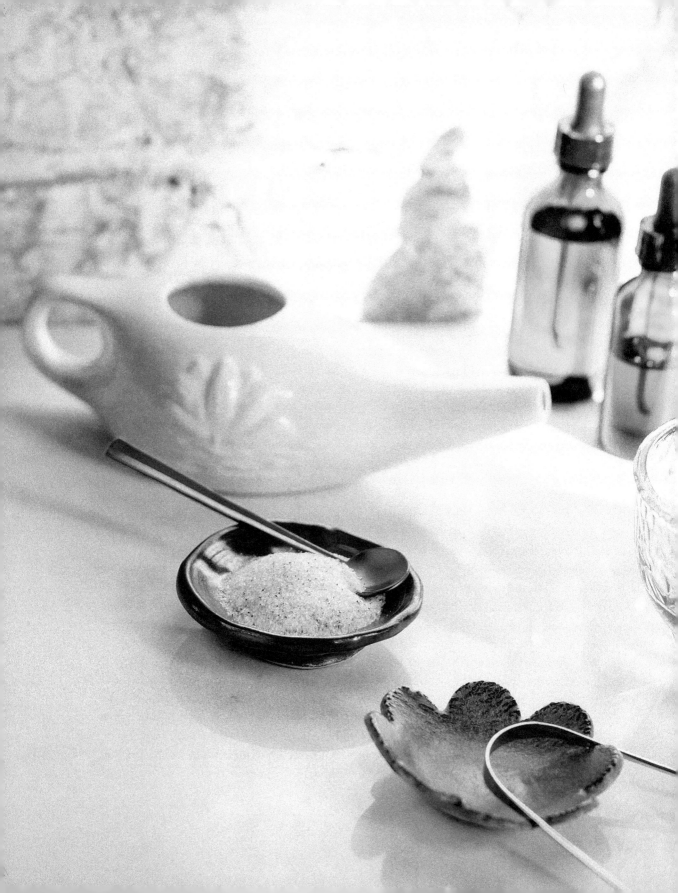

PART 1

Fundamentals of Health & Balance

Your body is speaking to you at every moment of every day. It is communicating each of its needs and challenges with simple, logical actions. Do you detect when your stomach tells you it is adequately full at each meal? Have you ever heard its tiny voice speaking to you, or do you just eat until discomfort arises and you feel heavy? Have you ever noticed the coating on your tongue when brushing your teeth? Did you know that the coating is your tongue revealing the state of your digestion, something that can help you decide which foods to eat each day? This is your body speaking in a language that most people have long forgotten, the innate wisdom that we all possess as infants but are not always encouraged to listen to as we grow into adults. The good news is that this language is easy to learn.

The colors and textures you see in your hair and skin when you peer into the mirror are hints of balance or imbalance. Your face—with its unique lines and creases, beauty marks and blemishes, and luster or lack thereof—tells a story of your health. Your eyes, often called the windows of the soul, share the truth of your being as emotions rise up and through them. Your tongue is a map of the internal world—the world of digestion, assimilation, and elimination. Your nails reveal secrets deep in your bones. Even your aches and pains are a cry: "Can you help? Here? There?" These are just some of the ways our bodies are always speaking to us.

Together, these bodily signs create a road map depicting the journey either away from balance or toward it. Before disease manifests, many road signs of warning may appear. Have you ever felt as if something in your body was just not right? Maybe you visited your doctor to report a series of seemingly unrelated symptoms, but the doctor found nothing wrong. These are the road signs. This is your intelligence speaking. Many ancient forms of medicine from India to China to Greece and beyond relied on reading and understanding these bodily signs to prevent and diagnose disease. If you are willing to look and listen carefully, you can understand your body's language and make prevention your key to health.

Ayurveda is a common-sense medicine we need in modern society. Originating more than 5,000 years ago in India, Ayurveda is a traditional medical science based on natural principles that apply to all life. It not only recognizes the uniqueness of each individual but also outlines principles that support better health for each body-mind type—the physiological and psychological characteristics of an individual that Ayurveda categorizes into three main types, which are described in detail in chapter 2. With the individual as its focus, Ayurveda offers a model of prevention-based medicine that many cultures lack today—a true system of health care, not just sick care! Although Ayurveda prioritizes self-observation and self-care practices to foster good health, Ayurveda also has many specialized branches such as internal medicine, surgery, pediatrics, psychology, and rejuvenation to improve health when we are sick or injured.

According to Ayurveda, health care has four simple steps.

1. Learn the basic principles that apply to all life, so that you can see yourself and the world around you clearly.

2. Use these principles to determine your body-mind type, and then follow diet and lifestyle practices appropriate for your type.

3. Learn to attune to the cycles of nature, living in harmony with the seasons and thus maximizing your energy.

4. Cleanse the body regularly and follow up with a period of rejuvenation to remove any unhealthy accumulation before it can develop into a problem.

Part I of this book walks you through these four steps; Part II lays out a simple 31-day protocol to prepare your body to go in to and ease out of a gentle Ayurvedic cleanse.

CHAPTER ONE

The Essence of Ayurveda

Intelligence is your birthright. Your body is a miracle, and every one of the trillions of cells working together in your body is intelligent. They all know exactly how to function, which nutrients to use, and how to cooperate with one another. Ayurveda, which translates as the "science of life," is based on a firm understanding of this intelligence, and the classic textbooks of Ayurveda state that disease often begins when we ignore the body's wisdom.

Your body is logical in every action and reaction, and it speaks out against any action that does not foster good health. Sometimes it speaks quietly, such as through a coating on your tongue, and other times it speaks loudly, for example, through the symptoms of a hangover. If you ignore this intelligence too long, it will eventually respond with "dis-ease." Disease is not a mysterious or instantaneous event; rather, it comes from a progression of imbalances that accumulate in a logical and natural order over time.

It is easier to care for one's health than to cure a disease. One of Ayurveda's goals, therefore, is to prevent disease by encouraging individuals to take personal responsibility for their health. A daily practice of caring for oneself as a good mother cares for her child—with healthy food, proper exercise, protection against the elements of nature, restful sleep, nurturing touch, and abundant love—is a big step toward ensuring a healthy body and mind. We each have a responsibility to be a good parent to ourselves so that we can contribute our best potential to our families, our communities, and the world.

Longevity

According to Ayurveda, the body is the vehicle for our energy, our minds, and even our souls. It is difficult to focus on anything else when the body is sick or experiencing pain. Like a wounded animal that instinctively hides to protect itself, we seek shelter when we are sick by turning inward to focus our energy on healing. If the body is not sound, there is little energy available for learning, creativity, growth, or transformation. Imbalance and illness limit our ability to expand our lives beyond our own immediate physical needs, and this limitation prohibits expansion of our minds, hearts, and spirits.

Longevity is one of Ayurveda's primary aims, so people have a lifetime of opportunity to develop a spiritual practice that takes them beyond the physical existence of the body. Ayurveda's goal is one hundred healthy years for each person. For many this goal may sound unrealistic, because many people now reach their eighties, nineties, or are even older, but most are not healthy. This does not need to be the case.

The process of aging is universal; we will all pass on from this life one day and most of us will grow old first. But the symptoms of "aging" have more to do with the relative state of balance in the body than with physical age. Dan Buettner, in collaboration with *National Geographic* and the National Institute on Aging, studied areas of the world where centenarians are common. In the book *Blue Zones: 9 Lessons For Living Longer from the People*

Who've Lived the Longest, he reported the common threads in communities where people live to age one hundred at a rate ten times greater than the global average, where life expectancy is typically twelve years longer than the worldwide average, and where the rate of middle-age mortality is a fraction of that in other places. He found diet and lifestyle factors to be the most substantial differences.

Genetics does play a role in the rate at which one's body shows signs of aging—some people have gray hair at age twenty, while others have a full head of dark hair at eighty—but it is not the only factor. The degenerative symptoms and diseases typically associated with old age can occur at a young age if the body is severely imbalanced. For example, arthritis of the hands is commonly seen in the elderly, but it could also manifest in a young person who uses his or her hands in a repetitive and excessive way, as a welder does. According to Ayurveda, the reverse is also true: The body can remain soft, supple, and flexible into old age when people perform proper self-care and maintenance throughout their lives.

Definition of Health

Health is a lot like a garden. The seeds of genetics and our natural intelligence carry our potential.

When planted in fertile soil with enough water and nutrients, good health sprouts. It requires the hard work of daily care and the diligence of maintenance to help it continue to grow into its fullness. Nature provides the setting and ingredients, but we must put forth the effort if we want to harvest the bounty of good health.

One obstacle to this bounty is that many cultures define "health" solely as the absence of disease. We all know long-term cigarette smokers, survivors of heart attacks, and individuals with diabetes who feel "healthy" despite obvious manifestations of disease. Conversely, many individuals feel "unhealthy" with unexplained symptoms of imbalance, but their doctors report them to be "normal." So what is health?

Ayurveda defines health in an extremely different way:

A person who has balanced physiological forces, balanced metabolic fire, properly formed tissues and waste products, who is established in Self, and whose being (mind-body-soul-senses) is full of bliss, is a healthy individual.

—translation from ***Charaka Samhita***, an ancient Ayurvedic textbook

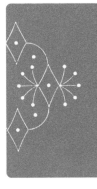

AYURVEDIC TOOLBOX: GET OUT

Observe: Cultivate the skill of observing qualities in yourselves and the environment.

Understand: Use the principles of Ayurveda to understand what these qualities mean for your body-mind type and current imbalance.

Transform: Make intelligent choices based on this knowledge to transform your health.

Twenty Qualities
— or ten pairs of opposites —

PAIRS	IN NATURE	IN THE BODY
Light/Heavy	dandelion seed/ boulder	underweight/ overweight
Sharp/Dull	thorn/mud	sharp pain/ dull sensation
Cold/Hot	winter/ summer	cold extremities such as hands or feet/fever
Dry/Oily	desert/ rain forest	dry/oily skin
Rough/ Smooth	bark/leaf	rough/ smooth nails or hair
Dense/ Liquiad; Amorphous	earth/water	muscles/blood
Hard/Soft	rocks/moss	bones/fat
Mobile/ Static; Stable	wind/earth	racing thoughts/ stable focus
Subtle (having little to no physical mass)/Gross (having solid bulk or physical mass)	air/wood	emotions/ flesh
Sticky/Clear	tree sap/air	mucus/ tears

This definition provides clear indicators of health. It offers criteria for measuring it and uplifts the truth that our natural state of health can bring bliss on all levels. Ayurveda is clear that health can be established only if it includes all aspects of ourselves—body, mind, soul, and senses. This is a rare jewel, but it is attainable.

Ayurveda provides a unique framework that is proactive, engaged, and tailored to the individual. It provides tools for self-assessment, systematic steps for cultivating health, and individual guidelines for maintaining it, based on three body-mind types. The steps to cultivate health can be summed up with three actions: observe, understand, transform. See the sidebar on page 13 for details.

Qualities

Every plant, every animal, and every substance on our planet has unique qualities. Water, for example, is cold unless heated by the sun or a fire. Water is heavy, and thus flows downward with gravity. Fire, on the other hand, is hot and light, and its flames flare upward. Each of these qualities exists as one of a pair of opposites: hot or cold, light or heavy, smooth or rough, moist or dry.

We are constantly using these pairs to maintain balance, or homeostasis, in our bodies. In the heat of summer we seek out a cool drink, a shady spot to sit, or a fan, because opposites balance each other. This is one of the first lessons we learn as infants. Even a young child learns to seek out the warmth of a mother's arms or a blanket when cold. This innate knowledge grows over time as we begin to understand the world around us, but the first step is learning to observe these qualities.

OBSERVATION WALK

Take a walk in nature and try to observe qualities in each unique element you notice. Bring the list of pairs on page 14 and make sure to find at least one example in nature of each quality. Start by describing the weather, the geography, and the season. Look at the trees: Describe their structure, bark, and leaves with these pairs of opposites. Notice that different species of trees have slightly different qualities. Observe the earth and any plants, bodies of water, and animals you encounter. Notice any qualities that are present in abundance in the area.

Finding Balance

The principle of opposites is constantly at play in nature: The cool of night follows the heat of day; a dry season follows the rainy season; and the cool of fall follows the heat of summer. These vacillations between opposite qualities create a natural rhythm that brings balance to the environment. All of the qualities manifest at a proper place and time.

Our bodies also have a natural rhythm. Each quality must exist in the proper amount for balance to exist. For example, the hot, sharp, and penetrating qualities of the digestive acids in your stomach require sufficient cool, oily, and sticky mucus to protect the lining of the stomach. If the proper balance is not maintained, an ulcer could result. All imbalances in the body follow a logical progression. In the case of an ulcer, you might first feel heat in the stomach, then a burning sensation or acid reflux, and if it continues for a long time, pain as the heating acids ultimately eat through the lining of the stomach. When the natural balance is disrupted, we must act.

If you are feeling hot, you can encourage a return to balance when you apply cold in any form,

such as exposure to a cold climate, cold foods or drinks; a cool shower or bath; an herb with cooling properties; or a cooling breath or yoga pose. We may have numerous options, because everything in the universe has qualities, so anything that has the cooling quality could be a potential medicine to restore balance. In the previous example of an ulcer, a cooling diet would help to soothe the burning heat in the stomach and restore balance, especially if someone adopts this diet at the first signs of heat.

Ayurveda uses this principle of opposites at every level of the body to maintain health. Every food and drink you consume has an effect on the body. Every thought and emotion you experience affects your body. Seasons and climates do as well. Exercise or lack of exercise, self-care or lack of self-care, and sleep or lack of sleep all have an impact. The universe is full of potential for healing. All we need to do is observe our predominant qualities, understand how they are affecting us, and transform ourselves by applying the principle of opposites. Ayurveda recognizes that each body is different, so the recipe for health it prescribes requires an individual analysis, which is explained in the next chapter.

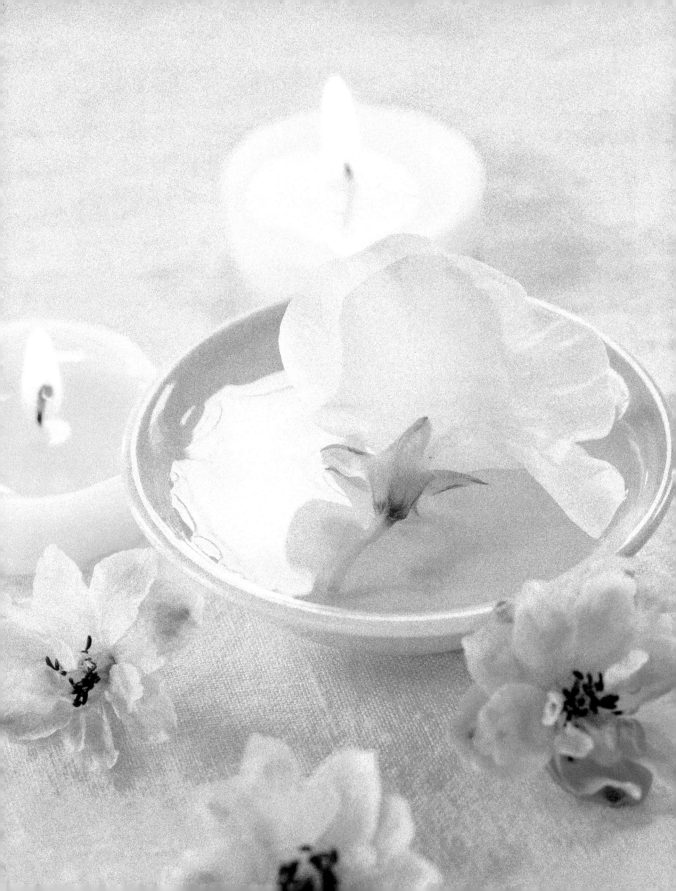

CHAPTER TWO

Understanding Your Body-Mind Type

Ayurveda uses this individuality as a basis for understanding health. Each of us requires different foods, exercises, activities, and daily practices to maintain health or restore it when we lose balance. Understanding your body-mind type can empower you to make choices every day to help improve your health even if you have a chronic condition.

Ancient seers, or *rishis*, observed nature and noticed that the human being is a microcosm of the macrocosm. The forces present in nature are parallel to forces that shape our internal universe. Three fundamental principles govern movement, structure, and transformation. The principle of movement is like a wind or breeze, the principle of structure is like earth, and the principle of transformation is like fire. These three principles are cogs in the machine of creation and in the body and mind. When they are associated with the internal organization of the body and mind we call them *doshas*. In Sanskrit, they are *Vata*, *Kapha*, and *Pitta*, respectively. For the purposes of this book, we will associate these principles with the body-mind types Breeze, Mountain, and Fire, respectively.

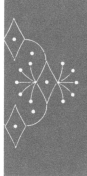
The dosha that is predominant in you creates your body-mind type. Predominance in Vata, or Breeze, creates a body-mind type that is mobile, variable, light like the wind, and as delicate as a flower. Predominance of Kapha, or Mountain, creates a body-mind type that is sturdy and strong like a mountain. Predominance of Pitta, or Fire, creates an individual who is active, driven, and full of fire and heat. Each of these three types possesses specific qualities and actions that distinguish them from one another, and they require different self-care routines.

Vata Dosha
- or the breeze type -

In Ayurveda, the internal principle of movement is called *vata dosha*, from the Sanskrit root *va* meaning "to move." It is a combination of all the qualities of space (ether) and air elements. Air moving through a space creates a wind. The central nervous system controls all internal movements, from the conscious contracting of muscles to the unconscious beating of the heart. Thus, vata dosha is intimately linked with the nervous system.

When predominant, vata will manifest a physical body that is light and thin with little fat stores. Because of this, and because fat in the form of

a myelin sheath is the insulator of every nerve fiber, the nervous system is not well insulated in vata-predominant individuals. This makes the vata individual particularly sensitive, like an exposed electrical wire. The Ayurvedic saying, "Treat a vata like a delicate flower" reflects this sensitivity.

Qualities

Cold, dry, light, rough, mobile, subtle, and sensitive are all qualities of the Breeze type, but the most pronounced is mobile. The dominant quality of Breeze is movement. Consider the incredibly vital role movement plays in our organisms: The constant and consistent movement of our hearts, breath, peristalsis, urine, sweat, lymphatic fluid, cellular respiration, blood, oxygen, nutrition into cells, waste out of cells, cerebrospinal fluid, thoughts, and attention all play nuanced, powerful roles in health. When this movement is natural, relaxed, regular, and flowing, we experience health. When it is too fast, too slow, or otherwise thwarted, we experience disturbance.

Our internal rhythms and movements track and respond to the external environment. To better understand this, picture a flower in bloom in a meadow. As the sun rises, her petals open in response. She turns toward the sun and follows it along its path across the sky. A gentle wind blows and she waves. Stronger winds blow and she bends. A bee lands on her, then later a butterfly. She is not only subjected to and affected by external movement but also to her own mobile responses to the environment. Her natural internal movement influences how she follows the path of the sun and opens and closes her petals; her internal responses to the interactions with the bee and the butterfly; and the flow of nutrients, sunlight, and waste throughout her organism.

Like the flower, we human beings are constantly in motion—a combination of our internal physiological motion and our responses to the environment. When the mobile quality is balanced, we can stay focused, have routine times for bowel habits, our heartbeats are regular, and other processes that motion governs are healthy. Although the mobile quality is a defining feature of Vata, the other qualities associated with this type tend to affect and afflict Breeze types also. They tend to be quite thin, due to the light quality; have dry or rough skin, bowels, and hair, due to the dry and rough quality; and have active imaginations and

inner lives, due to the subtle quality that creates an expansive mind.

Physical Constitution

An individual with a Breeze body type may be very tall or very short, thin, lanky, and sometimes has asymmetric features. The person's frame tends to be narrow, thin, and light, with a small bone structure, light muscle mass, and little body fat. The light and dry qualities of the Breeze keep these individuals thin despite how much food they eat, and it is often difficult for them to gain weight. Without much insulation, they can easily feel sensitive to cold, wind, dry weather, and even to too much stimulation from the environment or surroundings. Facial features are small, thin, or delicate, with quick or frequent movements such as blinking often. Their skin, hair, and nails may show signs of rough and dry qualities, and the qualities of mobility and variability are pronounced in most of their actions and preferences.

Nature

Because movement is the most distinguishing factor for this type, Breeze individuals move fast, walk fast, and talk fast. Like a little butterfly or a hummingbird, they move quickly from one thing to the next—ideas, thoughts, projects, conversations, and even relationships. They often enjoy a variety of physical and social activities, travel, and new experiences. Ideas and thoughts flow through their minds easily, like a constant wind giving them great creative powers. This expansive ability of the mind influences many Breeze types to become musicians, artists, or writers. It is often difficult for these individuals to slow down their bodies and minds, as this quality of mobility permeates their lives and their love of variability may keep them from establishing solid, lasting routines.

Kapha Dosha
— *or the mountain type* —

Kapha is the Ayurvedic term used to describe the physiological principles of structure and lubrication considered the body's glue, or cohesive force. The solid structures of the body such as bones, joints, muscles, and fat, as well as the liquid or lubricating substances such as saliva, mucus, plasma, lymph, and synovial fluid in the joints are composed of the building blocks of kapha. The word *kapha* translates as "that which flourishes by water" or "that which holds things together."

Qualities

The qualities of the earth element—hard, dense, solid, and stable—combined with the qualities of water element—liquid, soft, fluid, and cold—describe all of the body's physical structures, from bones and muscles to lymph and plasma. An individual who has a predominance of the kapha dosha will have abundant body mass and lubrication, which form a strong, solid structure not easily disturbed by external forces, much like a mountain.

Think of the qualities of a majestic mountain: large, solid, stable, heavy, dense, and hard. The mountain seems immovable. Does the wind change the mountain at all? Yes, but not the way it affects a flower. We know that mountains move and change over time, but gradually. The forces of nature erode a mountain, but it takes thousands of years. Now picture the mountain more closely; imagine a stream trickling from the cloud-covered top and meandering down through cold, mossy rocks. Consider the qualities you see here: moist, smooth, soft, cold, and slow. All of the qualities listed for both the sturdy earth and softer water elements compose the Mountain body type.

Physical Constitution

The physical constitution of a Mountain is large, solid, and stable, with good strength, stamina, and resilience. The Mountain's bone structure, muscle mass, and store of body fat are larger than that of the other body types, and the incredible insulation this creates makes the Mountain seem barely affected by heat or cold, hunger or thirst, and even lack of sleep or excessive activity. People with this body type move slowly in all aspects of their lives and enjoy the comfort of routines that are reliably stable and long lasting. The heaviness and inertia they can accumulate tend to make change and variability challenging. A slower metabolism makes it easy for them to store up excesses but difficult to lose weight or clear out accumulations, such as mucus. Their facial features are large and broad, with smooth, moist skin, abundant long eyelashes, full lips, and a thick, luxurious head of hair. They are sturdy and stable in their physical bodies and in their routines, thoughts, and emotions.

Nature

The nature of the Mountain type is to hold. They physically hold on to more muscle mass, weight, and

MOUNTAIN TYPE

Actions: structure and lubrication

Elements: earth and water

Qualities: cool, moist, heavy, stable, smooth, oily, dense, liquid, hard, soft, gross, dull, and sticky

Body frame: large, heavy, and dense

Movements: slow and steady

moisture than other types do, but they also excel at holding on to money, relationships, and love. Their reliable, steady emotions make them wonderful friends, confidants, and teachers, able to offer sympathy and empathy with ease and bring comfort to others. Comfort plays a key role in their lives, especially at home—where they often like to stay, enjoying the leisure of reading, cooking, or relaxing. A lavishly comfortable bed, sitting area, or car may be a sign of the Mountain type. Strong memory is another asset of the Mountain even though this type may take longer than others to learn or gather information. Like elephants, Mountains "never forget," which serves them well in the academic and business worlds but can be challenging in their personal and emotional lives, because they may hold on to old emotions, experiences, and grudges. When they are balanced, they can easily forgive and lavish love.

The Mountain and the Breeze look like opposites in most ways: One is rarely affected by the external environment, the other constantly overwhelmed by it; one is immovable or slow, the other is in constant motion and fast. The two types share one major quality: cold. Neither the Breeze nor the Mountain generates heat; their nature is cool.

Pitta Dosha
— or the fire type —

The center of our solar system is the intensely hot star we call the sun; the center of a cell is a metabolic command center called the nucleus; and the center of the human body holds the acids and digestive enzymes we call our digestive fire, or *agni*. Fire in all its forms is the universal principle that creates transformation. The ancient Ayurvedic rishis clearly perceived this transformational internal force

and named it *pitta* from the root verb *tapa* meaning "to heat."

Qualities

Pitta dosha combines qualities of the fire element with qualities of the water element, resulting in a combination of qualities: oily, sharp, hot, light, spreading, and liquid. Pitta is present in the stomach region for transformation of food and in the brain to transform stimuli from the sense organs into thoughts, feelings, and emotions. Each cell must have adequate pitta to carry out cellular metabolism and direct proper functioning of its parts. A pitta-predominant individual will exhibit this fire in all areas of the physical body and the mind.

The Fire type, unlike the Breeze and Mountain types, is inherently hot. Picture yourself sitting next to a roaring campfire as it lights up and warms the surrounding area. Observe the continuous movement. Notice how easily the flames build and spread, transforming the wood and everything it touches. Know that if you touch its flame you, too, will feel the fire's sharp bite.

Physical Constitution

The Fire type is medium in size and build: medium height, muscle mass, and amount of body fat. The face has sharp, medium-size features. The manifestations of Fire characteristics are visible everywhere on the body. The skin is sensitive to the sun, fair, freckled, and slightly oily. The cheeks are rosy, the lips are red, and a brightness or lightness illuminates the eyes. The internal heat of transformation keeps the Fire type's body and mind hot, even in a cold season or climate. The digestive fire is strong, allowing Fire individuals to eat heartily without gaining unneeded weight.

Nature

The mind of a Fire individual mirrors a strong appetite. People with this body type have a passion for knowledge, experience, and intensity. Fire is a transformative force, and in their mind it creates a sharp intellect with a desire for understanding. The questions of why and how are of utmost importance. Their sharp minds naturally create order and organization, allowing them to see patterns and big pictures, be detail-oriented (sometimes to the point of perfectionism), and good at strategizing and coordinating when they are in balance. The Fire type is the epitome of Type A personality in our multitasking culture. This fire can fuel mental activities and work, intense physical activities (like skydiving, rock climbing, or running a marathon), and passionate emotions. The fiery emotions of frustration, anger, and rage can flare up when the Fire is out of balance. Burnout can also be a real consequence of an imbalance of too much intensity or activity.

Now the important question remains: Which type are you? A Breeze, a Fire, or a Mountain? You will most likely see in yourself aspects of all three types, because we must have all three natural forces to exist. Still, most of us have a strong tendency toward one or two of these categories. According to Ayurveda, each person, from the moment of birth, is a unique combination of these three forces. The resulting combination is known as one's "constitution." Although most people have a strong predominance in one or two of the three doshas, an individual may have all three in equal amount. Each type has its strengths and weaknesses, and the foundation of health lies in knowing your personal combination.

The word *dosha* actually translates as "that which goes out of balance," which describes the aspect we often see most clearly. For this reason, Ayurveda seeks to first determine your constitution, called *prakriti*, and then your current state of imbalance, called *vikriti*.

DELICATE YET STRONG

People with a predominance of Fire encounter unique circumstances that the other two types do not. Although their intellectual abilities and ambitions are especially strong, their physical constitution can be somewhat delicate. For example, though competitive and slow to admit or even recognize it, they will indeed tire from strong physical labor more quickly than the Mountain type—especially if they are laboring in hot weather. The Fire type tends to identify with the strength of their own intellect and ambitions and may believe they are also physically strong. Because they respect their ambitions and intellect more than their body, they often pursue their ambitions despite their body telling them for years that it can't keep up. It is not uncommon for the Fire type to disbelieve or ignore the delicacy of their physical constitution until it screams at them, forcing them to slow down. It is therefore a good practice for Fire types to surrender to the pace of their bodies—a practice that does not come easily—if they want to maintain physical health as well as intellectual prowess. This first requires that they are in touch with the real pace of their body, which requires a practice of internal reflection. —*DR. CLAUDIA WELCH*

FIRE TYPE

Action: transformation

Elements: fire and water

Qualities: hot, light, sharp, mobile, liquid, and spreading

Body frame: medium

Movements: moderate pace and deliberate

Filling out the Constitution Checklist on page 138 is one way to determine which doshas are predominant for you. Clear observation is the first step. This requires an honest assessment of your qualities, a process that can be difficult at first. It may be helpful to fill out the checklist with a friend or family member who can give you perspective. The checklist covers physical attributes of your body, mental tendencies, likes and dislikes, and even emotional patterns. If you find that you have a combination of qualities from more than one type for one category, mark each one. For example, if your skin is both dry and fair, then place a check next to each statement. The goal is to find an overall trend, though many people have a sense of their type before they go through the list. When you finish, total the number of checks in each category to see where your predominance resides.

Sometimes it is helpful to answer the Constitution Checklist from the perspective of your childhood, given that your constitution is the unique combination of these doshas at the moment of your birth. Occasionally, our true nature is masked by the imbalances we have accumulated over the years.

Take your time when filling out the Constitution Checklist. Consider your characteristics as a whole throughout your lifetime. If you find that your answers are dramatically different from the answers you would give based on your childhood self, create two columns and answer one for each, to see how they compare.

The Breeze
— in and out of balance —

The strengths of any body-mind type are present when an individual is in balance, and the weaknesses show up when she is out of balance. The Breeze individual exhibits creativity, clarity, imagination, and love of diversity when in balance. Healthy functions encompass all conscious and unconscious movements in the body, as well as all muscular movements, as described here:

- Inward movement or intake: sensory stimuli, mental processes, inhalation, and swallowing;

- Upward movement: exhalation, coughing, speaking/expression, hiccuping, and vomiting;

- Digestive movement: coordinating the process of digestion and movement through the digestive tract;

- Circulatory movement: heart pulsation, movement of blood, and lymphatic movement; and

- Downward movement: elimination of wastes and reproductive fluids, expelling the fetus, and grounding.

These movements are all necessary to keep the body at optimum health, and, when in balance, the Breeze individual experiences each type of movement in proper proportions.

When Breeze individuals are out of balance, the natural predominant qualities—cold, light, dry, rough, mobile, subtle, and clear—will accumulate. This means someone may feel internally cold, have cold extremities, and could develop an aversion to wind or cold. Signs of imbalance manifest as dark discolorations of the body or wastes, such as in the eyes, nails, skin, urine, or feces. Skin, hair, nails, lips, mouth, nose, eyes, ears, joints, or the colon may become dry, because these are parts of the body that require fluids and mucus to function properly.

For example, synovial fluid in the joints is the natural lubrication that eases movement, and when the dry quality affects these fluids, one can hear cracking and popping sounds with joint movement. If that persists for some time, pain and discomfort may follow, eventually limiting the range of motion in the joint and possibly creating deformities in its shape and structure. If the dry quality affects the colon, the mucus lining will lose its natural lubrication and the stools will become hard, leading to constipation.

Excessive mobility can lead to muscular twitches, spasms, irregular bowel movements, or a busy or scattered mind that cannot stop, even to sleep (insomnia). Accumulation of vata in the colon, considered its homesite in the body, can contribute to constipation, pain in the low back, hips, or thighs, eventually leading to sciatica. The variability or weakness of digestive strength produces gas, bloating, and other kinds of abdominal discomfort. Too much lightness can manifest as insomnia, a light-headed or ungrounded feeling, anxiety, or nervousness. Emotionally, an imbalance can also create fear, instability, or insecurity. Throughout the book, we categorize all of these as Breeze imbalances.

The Mountain
— in and out of balance —

Strong, sturdy Mountain individuals are grounded, loving, compassionate, and reliable when in balance, making them good teachers and caregivers. Healthy functions include providing raw materials that build all the tissues of the body and lubricate or insulate these parts of the body:

- Stomach: to aid digestion;

- Lungs and heart: to reduce friction from the constant movement of these organs and counteract the dryness of the air we breathe;

- Joints: to allow fluid movements;

- Mouth: to allow taste by the tongue, the act of swallowing, and the start of the process of digestion; and

- Brain and nervous system: to produce the cerebrospinal fluid, the myelin sheath, and white matter of the brain

We need adequate substance to build and maintain all body tissue, to lubricate the body and ensure ease of movement, and to protect the tissues and organs from damage. When in balance, the Mountain easily supplies the proper amount of materials for each function and gives strength to the body.

When out of balance, the Mountain individual's natural qualities—cool, heavy, smooth, oily, dense, liquid, soft, dull, stable, gross, and sticky—will create excess accumulations in the body and mind. In the body, heaviness, weight gain, lethargy, fluid retention, edema, or nausea may manifest. A Mountain imbalance might be more noticeable during a woman's menses, when all of those symptoms may affect her at the same time. A dull or cool digestive fire can create slow digestion or allow excess mucus to accumulate in the lungs, sinuses, stools, or stomach, which is considered the homesite of kapha in the body. Thick, white accumulations or discharges show imbalance, and accumulations of soft or hard masses such as fatty tumors, cysts, and cancerous or benign growths are common. Emotionally, the excess stable quality may turn into attachment, stubbornness, or greed when imbalanced.

As an example of how imbalance progresses, dull digestive fire could lead to overproduction of mucus in the stomach, creating nausea and a feeling of heaviness. These symptoms might lead a Mountain individual to rest in the daytime instead of being physically active—activity is important to counteract their stability and density. The accumulation might extend to the lungs, where it reduces the intake of oxygen and energy, creating lethargy and more inactivity, which may eventually result in weight gain, fluid retention, swollen joints, and the inability of the body to efficiently rid itself of wastes. This may also affect a person's emotional health, creating a sense of depression. Throughout the book, we categorize these as Mountain imbalances.

THE HOUSE OF THE BODY

Imagine building a house:

Kapha (Mountain) functions as the principle of **structure and stability** and supplies the raw materials to build the foundation, structure, walls, floors, insulation, and every fixture and feature of the house. In the body, the gross physical components are bones, muscles, fat, organs, and fluids. Building a house or a body requires gross, physical "stuff," and the qualities of the Mountain type reflect this.

Pitta (Fire) is the heating system of the house and the body. The fire in the kitchen's stove transforms raw materials of food into easily digested meals, just as the fire in the belly is responsible for internal transformation of various foods into a substance that can nourish every cell of the body. Pitta is the principle providing for both **temperature regulation and transformation.** In the house, the heating system consists of a source and pipes—not as much physical stuff, but extremely important to the house. The qualities of the Fire type are subtler in nature than the Mountain's qualities.

Vata (Breeze) is the electrical system, which resembles the sensory impulses and the nervous system in our bodies where all **movement** originates. Its qualities are the most subtle and mobile in the house.

From the gross to the subtle, all parts of the house are equally important, just as the three doshas are needed in the body in the proper proportion.

The Fire
— in or out of balance —

The positive qualities associated with a Fire individual who is in balance are organization, order, clear communication, and a sharp intellect. Healthy functions are related to temperature regulation and transformation: transformation of food into energy, data into information, information into wisdom, and raw elements into biologically refined substances that nourish the body. These functions are particularly active in these parts of the body:

- Stomach and small intestines (considered the homesite of pitta in the body), as digestive enzymes;

- Liver, as bile;

- Skin, for temperature regulation;

- Eyes, for visual perception; and

- Heart-mind, for digestion of sensory input into thoughts, feelings, and emotions.

When the Fire is in balance, proper amounts of heat, acids, and enzymes are present to carry out natural functions.

When out of balance, the heating qualities of the Fire start to consume the body and mind. Hot or burning sensations, redness, inflammation, yellow discolorations, and sharp sensations of pain can manifest anywhere in the body, including the eyes, stomach, and joints. The stools may become soft or liquid and dark yellow in color. The yellow discoloration of eyes, nails, teeth, skin, or any other body part or waste product reflects an imbalance. The skin may become sensitive and prone to inflammation, resulting in acne, hives, or rashes. Digestive issues include loose stools, acid reflux, heartburn, gastritis, gastric ulcers, pain, or burning sensations. Fire individuals may experience excessive thirst, and the heated emotions of anger, frustration, rage, and jealousy may flare up. Throughout the book, we categorize these as Fire imbalances.

After you have filled out the Constitution Checklist (see page 138), fill out the Imbalance Checklist (see page 139). Answer according to how you are feeling **in this moment**—not your past history or your overall trends. This will give you more-accurate information on your current state of imbalance. The imbalance that you are experiencing may or may not be similar to your constitution. An individual with a Breeze constitution may easily be swayed into a Breeze imbalance, because they already have an abundance of those qualities, but that is not always the case. A person with a Breeze constitution can have a Mountain imbalance from having a sedentary lifestyle over a period of years. A person with a Fire constitution could "blow out" their fire from too much activity or movement, resulting in a Breeze imbalance—or that same excessive movement could "ignite an inferno," resulting in a Fire imbalance. It is important to accurately discern both constitution and imbalance separately.

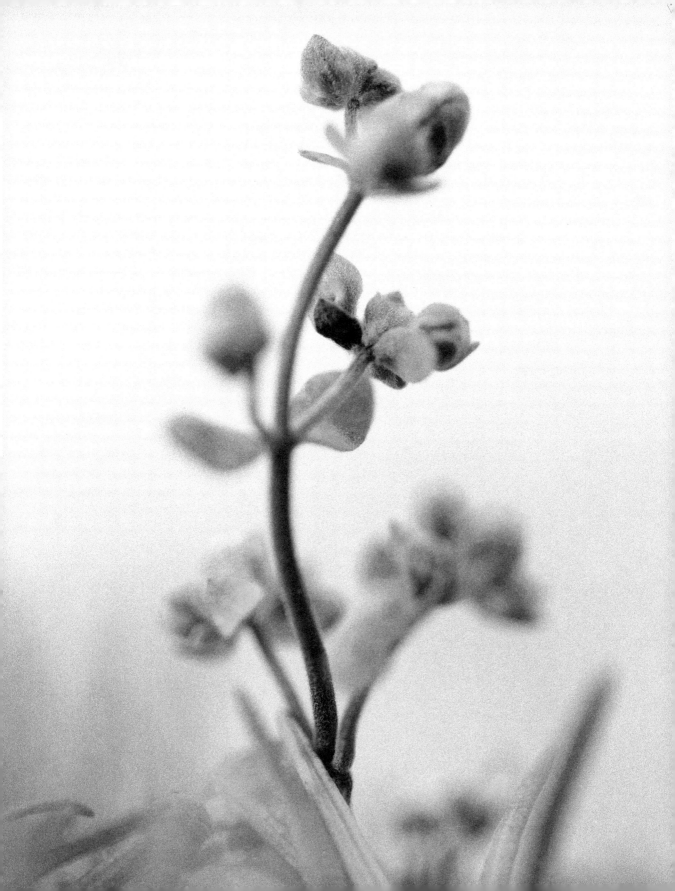

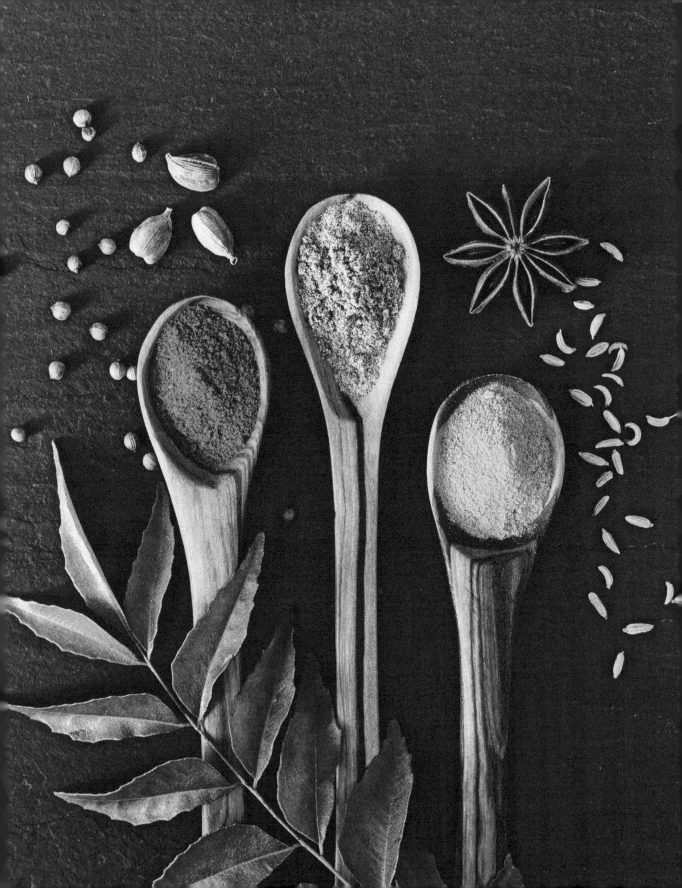

"Let food be thy medicine, and medicine be thy food."

—Hippocrates, Father of Modern Medicine

CHAPTER THREE

Foods for Balance

Personal transformation begins with knowledge. You have observed yourself and your natural qualities, filled out the Constitution Checklist and Imbalance Checklist (see pages 138 and 139) to determine and understand your unique body-mind type and imbalance, and now you are ready to make choices that can transform your health. Food can, and should be medicine—this has been the basis of most health-care systems throughout time. Dr. Mark Hyman, in a TED talk on functional medicine, states that poor lifestyle choices, including diet, cause the majority of chronic, degenerative diseases, making them preventable. That means millions of individuals could have avoided suffering if they had the knowledge to transform themselves with their choices and acted on it. Luckily, you can gain this knowledge and transform yourself and your health. Are you ready to start?

Food-Medicine

Understanding what qualities are in the foods you eat is essential for health. Food builds every cell of your body. What you eat is without a doubt one of the most important decisions you make every day, though no single diet is right for every person. Ayurveda has pointed out two simple principles you can use to determine which foods are appropriate for you: the "principle of opposites" and "like increases like." These principles are two sides of the same coin: Similar qualities increase and opposite qualities decrease.

In general, we want to eat foods that have qualities opposite of those qualities that are high in our bodies. For example, if I feel too heavy, I want foods that are light in quality. If I feel too hot, I want cooling foods. Whatever type you are, you will tend to have an excess of that type's qualities. For example, the Breeze individual is cold, dry, and light in nature and therefore finds comfort and balance eating warm, moist, and heavy foods. The Mountain is cold, heavy, and moist in nature and needs foods that are hot, light, and dry to help bring balance. Finally, the Fire individual exhibits hot and light

qualities and finds balance when eating foods that are cool and heavy. And though your constitution has a bit of each type, by following a diet designed for your predominant type, you can improve your balance and health. Like increases like, so if you are already cold and you eat ice cream, the logical effect is that you get colder. We can use this principle— and the principle of opposites—to make good decisions about our diet every day.

Whenever you eat something, the qualities in that food permeate your body. When you eat a chili pepper, the sharp, hot qualities first hit the tongue, then a burning sensation happens in your throat and stomach, and finally sweat begins to pour off of your brow. The heat of the pepper transfers to your being; you become hot like the pepper. To the Breeze individual, who is sensitive and delicate like a flower, this chili pepper might feel painful and overwhelming to the senses. To the sturdy, well-insulated Mountain, however, it might feel like a mild warming action that is a welcome change from his natural cool state. To a Fire type, the stimulation and rush of endorphins that follow might be exhilarating, but the stomach and digestive tract may continue to burn for days afterward. Food

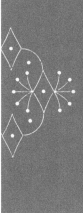

POTENCY OF FOODS

Ayurveda classifies each food by its heating or cooling influence on the body. With some sensitivity or practice of awareness, you can feel this potency, or *virya*, in the stomach. The term *virya* can also be translated as "strength," "energy," or "power." The potency of some foods can be easily discerned, such as with a cucumber, which feels cool and juicy in the mouth as well as the stomach. But some foods might be harder to "feel"—some grains, for example, are heating and some are cooling. A foods list can initially help give you some perspective, but ideally you will learn to listen to your body and feel for yourself. Check out Dr. Vasant Lad's *Ayurveda: The Science of Self-Healing* for a detailed foods list.

chosen with awareness can be medicine, but food chosen without awareness can be poison.

The Six Tastes

You can see the importance of observing two sets of qualities: those that are increased in you and those inherent in your food choices. Once again, the Ayurvedic tool to get you *out* of old habits and into new, healthier ones relies on observation. We also have another sense that helps us with the important job of choosing foods to be our medicine: taste.

Nature has designed a simple system of tastes to help us understand which foods will benefit us. According to Ayurveda, food has six tastes: sweet, sour, salty, pungent, bitter, and astringent. Each taste has one or more specific actions on the body, in addition to the heating or cooling effect initially felt on the tongue and in the stomach.

Sweet taste is present in fruits and some vegetables such as carrots and beets; in concentrated form in honey and sugar; and more subtly in grains, particularly rice. **Sour** shows up in citrus fruits or unripe berries and in fermented items like vinegar, yogurt, hard cheeses, and cultured or pickled vegetables. **Salty** taste is naturally inherent in seaweed and all varieties of salt. **Pungent**, also called "spicy," is the heating sensation from garlic, onions, peppers, and spices such as black pepper, chili pepper, and paprika. **Bitter** is the flavor of dark leafy greens. It is present to some degree in all green vegetables, but is also the roasted flavor we love in dark chocolate and coffee. Finally, **astringent** is a drying feeling in your mouth as if all of the saliva had evaporated. It is in pomegranates, unripe bananas, some beans, and some leafy greens, such as Swiss chard and spinach.

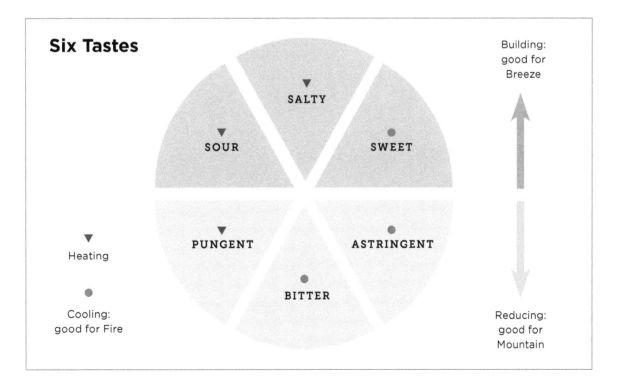

Six Tastes

SALTY

SOUR

SWEET

PUNGENT

ASTRINGENT

BITTER

Building: good for Breeze

Heating

Cooling: good for Fire

Reducing: good for Mountain

The sweet taste is heavy and cooling in nature and builds up the tissues of the body. The sour taste is heavy, moist, and heating in nature, but also builds up the tissues and adds bulk to the body. The salty taste is heating and helps to hold moisture in the body, so it also aids in creating more bulk by retaining water. The pungent taste is strongly heating, and this helps to create movement, melts cold accumulations, and burns up waste products. Bitter and astringent tastes, which are both light and cooling, aid the body in breaking down accumulations and tissues. Astringent reduces moisture. In a nutshell, sweet, sour, and salty tastes build tissues, and pungent, bitter, and astringent tastes break down tissues. We all need both building and breaking down to happen every day as old cells constantly break down (catabolic activity) and must be replaced by new ones (anabolic activity). Nevertheless, certain individuals need more of one action and less of the other.

Discerning the Six Tastes

Even though your body instinctively knows what to do with each taste, that does not mean that your mind necessarily understands the tastes and can discern them. It may take time to train your mind to understand and distinguish each taste. I suggest saying the word aloud as you taste it, to develop a strong association.

The sweet, sour, and salty tastes may be the easiest for you to discern if the bulk of your diet consists of fast foods, packaged foods, and processed foods, which rely heavily on these three tastes. Bitter and astringent are the tastes that are commonly lacking in our modern diet. Tasting bitter greens, green tea, or a bitter gourd (a green, bumpy vegetable sold in Indian markets) will help you to make the connection between mind and tongue. Bitter

and astringent tastes are often together in foods, particularly in foods we consider medicinal herbs, so it may be hard to separate them at first. Use a green unripe banana to discover the astringent taste alone without an excessively bitter taste.

Food Basics for Breeze Types

The light, cold, and dry Breeze individuals, who need more mass, insulation, and moisture, will benefit from eating more foods that are sweet, sour, and salty. These tastes give their bodies the adequate building blocks to create more muscle, store more adipose (fat) tissue, and retain more water.

Ideal foods for the Breeze type are warm—both in temperature and nature—moist, oily, nourishing, and well cooked. Cooking is a way of predigesting foods to increase the chances of proper digestion and make the nutrients more bioavailable. This is helpful for the often delicate and always variable digestive fire of the Breeze. Heavier foods like proteins, dairy, fats, and whole grains are all good for an individual with this constitution, to build healthy muscle and fat stores for strength and insulation. This is particularly true if the choices are also warming in nature, to counter the cold quality that predominates in the Breeze individual.

Chicken, turkey, eggs, or beef, in addition to easily digested legumes like mung beans, are good choices of protein. All dairy is good, particularly yogurt, buttermilk, or kefir, because these are warming in nature due to fermentation. A proper amount of healthy fat is essential in the form of warming oils, animal fats, or ghee. The best whole grain choices are basmati rice, brown rice, or oats. Vegetables and fruits should be well cooked, because raw foods can be hard for a weak digestive fire to process fully. If you are vegetarian or vegan, you can easily find

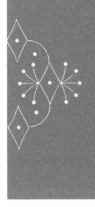
heavy, naturally sweet grains, vegetables, nuts, and beans that can nourish you as well as meat or dairy can. The best vegetables for Breeze individuals are heavy, sweet, and warming, such as root vegetables—specifically carrots, beets, and yams. Sweet, juicy fruits such as berries, mangoes, cherries, and bananas are ideal. For a complete list of "Eat More" foods, see page 78. It is important to keep in mind that even though dense, heavy, naturally sweet foods like dairy and some meats benefit Breeze individuals, because they have delicate digestive systems, portions should be small.

Mountain Basics

To stay in balance, the Mountain has markedly different food requirements than the Breeze has. Individuals who already have abundant moisture and a heavy build do not need to eat as many foods from the sweet, sour, and salty categories. Even a moderate amount of heavy, sweet grains; sour, juicy fruits; or salt may cause them to gain weight or swell from excessive water retention. The Mountain needs the three remaining tastes: pungent, bitter, and astringent. Foods with these tastes, particularly vegetables, are lighter and will increase the

Mountain's ability to break down old tissues and remove excess fluids.

Foods that are warm, dry, light, rough, spicy, and heating in nature are best for this type. Cooking foods also aids the Mountain types in proper digestion, because they often have a cool, dull, or slow digestive fire. Abundant vegetables are required for the bulk of their diet if this type is to remain healthy. Many vegetables are light in nature and packed with nutrients, minerals, phytochemicals, and energy, so the Mountain can meet most nutritional requirements by eating a wide variety of vegetables. They need limited grains, fats, and protein in their diet, to prevent excess heaviness, weight gain, or fluid retention. Avoiding or limiting all dairy, animal products, and most sweeteners is best for their health. Fruits are better for the Mountain when dried.

Light grains such as millet, amaranth, and corn are good choices. Plant-based proteins are lighter, with less fat; legumes, fermented soy products such as tempeh, or light seeds such as pumpkin and sunflower are healthy options. All vegetables are good except the sweet, juicy, or slimy ones, for example, sweet potato, cucumbers, or okra, respectively, and it is usually better to eat them cooked rather than raw. In moderation, dried apricots, cranberries, figs, and raisins are good fruits for the Mountain. Only honey or minimally processed or homegrown stevia (see page 34) should be used as sweeteners—and in small amounts. The Mountain type should use oils sparingly. For a complete list of "Eat More" foods, see page 101.

Fire Basics

The Fire type needs the three tastes that are cooling in nature—sweet, bitter, and astringent—for the bulk of their diet. The cooling nature of these flavors balances the natural heat of the Fire type.

A strong appetite and sharp digestive fire encourage Fire individuals to eat heartily. It is important that they eat enough heavy, nourishing foods that they can make it from one meal to the next without becoming *hangry*—the angry, irritable feeling that arises in a Fire individual when her previous meal has been digested and the strong digestive juices in her stomach are now beginning to eat away at her, potentially triggering her to lash out at anyone or anything that adds even the slightest amount

of irritation to her mounting hunger. (Although *hangry* may not be in the dictionary, many people relate to the feeling.) The entire nervous system can be agitated when the Fire individual does not eat enough food, and heat will rise, physically and emotionally, creating more Fire imbalance. This makes cooling foods that nourish and sustain important staples for the Fire types.

A diet consisting mostly of cooling fruits, vegetable, grains, legumes, or animal proteins (if you consume them) nuts, seeds, sweeteners, and minimal amounts of fats or oils typically serves a Fire individual well. Fruits that are juicy and cooling include avocadoes, apples, melons, grapes, pears, and figs. Green vegetables such as leafy greens, broccoli, zucchini, peas, green beans, and cucumbers are the most cooling. Nourishing grains include basmati rice, oats, wheat, and barley. All legumes are good protein options, as are cooling nuts and seeds such as coconut, almond, pumpkin, and sunflower. Sweet dairy such as milk and ghee are more cooling than fermented forms are. If you eat meat, chicken, turkey, and venison are the best options for the Fire individual, and you can use coconut, sunflower, safflower, and olive oils regularly in moderation. Raw foods are often appropriate for Fire individuals, because their sharp digestive fire can often handle the rough, cold, and hard qualities of those foods. For a complete list of "Eat More" foods, see page 120.

Spice-Medicines

Spices are concentrated food-medicines that display the six tastes in a stronger form than most foods do. Relative to other foods, only a small amount of a spice is required to have an effect on the tongue or the body. Cinnamon is sweet, pungent, bitter, and astringent in taste, and it makes a delicious condiment for sweet grains or cooked fruits. However, if you try to eat a spoonful, you may start to choke due to the strong astringent quality that dries up the secretions in your mouth and throat upon contact. Drawing on cinnamon's astringency, you could use it to dry up the excess secretions produced during a cold by making a tea and drinking it frequently. Regular consumption of cinnamon in foods and drinks could be a preventive measure for Mountain types, to reduce accumulation of mucus. Conversely, a dry Breeze individual might

SHARP DIGESTIVE FIRE

Just because the Fire type enjoys a sharp digestive fire, that may not always be healthy. If the liquid component of pitta increases too much, this can weaken a person's digestive power and lead to loose stools. If you find you cannot miss a meal, you need to eat, but you have loose stools, ulcers, or gastritis and are not digesting your food well, you may want to consult with your personal health care practitioner for more tailored recommendations.
—DR. CLAUDIA WELCH

try to limit use of this spice to ensure that adequate moisture remains in the body for lubrication.

Before the modern convenience of refrigeration, humans relied on spices for their preservative qualities as well as for their digestive and health-enhancing properties. Spices that healed wounds, prevented illness, and eased discomforts were a part of the home apothecary. People used ginger in steam to clear the sinuses of mucus or applied it to the body as a poultice, to ease stiffness of muscles and joints. They used cardamom, cinnamon, black pepper, and garlic internally to prevent colds and flus, and coriander tea as a wash for the eyes, to reduce inflammation. Turmeric acted as a natural antibiotic. Nutmeg with its astringent qualities could stop diarrhea.

Ayurveda still regards the kitchen as the medicine cabinet. Spices certainly can make food more delicious, but individual spices used at the right times by the right individual can also be medicinal. As with food, individuals should choose a spice based on their constitution, their imbalance, or the season to benefit from the spice's health-enhancing effects.

In general, to stimulate appetite, improve digestion, warm the body, dispel gas or bloating, and improve circulation, Breeze individuals do well with sweet, warming spices that are not overly heating. Ginger, hing, cardamom, and tulsi, also known as holy basil, are good examples. Keep in mind that spices that are too heating can dry the tissues, so although the warmth of some spices is good for Breeze types, they should avoid eating an excessive amount of hot, spicy foods. The Mountain, on the other hand, may do well with strong, hot, stimulating spices that build heat, create movement, dry up accumulations, and dispel stagnation—spices such as black pepper, paprika, garlic, cinnamon, and ginger. The Fire needs spices that can improve digestion (without adding excess heat), reduce inflammation, and cool the mind and heart, such as coriander, cumin, fennel, turmeric, and rose. The "Eat More" lists in chapters 6 through 8 can help you understand which foods, tastes, and spices to choose regularly for better health. Spices appropriate for your type also make your food easier to digest, and Ayurveda regards this as extremely important.

EAT FOR THE SEASON OR FOR YOUR IMBALANCE?

When we are in a relative state of balance, the foods that nature provides in each season will likely help us maintain that balance. Once we have gone out of balance, however, we need to observe a diet that will counter the heightened qualities in us, regardless of season. Following a diet specific for your predominant imbalance will be required for a time until you come back to health. Once imbalance symptoms disappear, follow a seasonal diet while always being aware of your constitutional needs.

The seasons each resemble one of the three doshas. Spring, at least in many locations, is cool and wet, with cloudy, heavy, and rainy days that result in sticky, slimy, and muddy earth—all the qualities associated with the Mountain type or kapha dosha. In summer, the days grow warm, then hot; moisture wanes and the long, bright days are full of activity and movement as the season of growth bursts wide open; this is like the heat and transformation of Fire type or pitta dosha. In autumn, days grow colder,

the air is dry, and vegetation dries up, increasing the Breeze qualities or vata dosha. In winter, cold accumulates and, depending on where you are, either dryness accumulates or it is very wet, increasing either Mountain or Breeze qualities. But in either case, we return again to the spring, when the frozen elements of winter melt and begin to flow again.

Spring season starts with tiny green shoots—the first of the year—that are bitter, astringent, or pungent in taste. Foods with these tastes provide a natural cleansing action to remove the accumulated stores from the winter and a heating action that counters the cold moistness from the environment. Eating an abundance of these foods is appropriate for most of us in the spring.

The summer brings more activity and more warmth in which sweet berries and fruits can grow, along with the first of the light summer vegetables, including leafy greens. These foods are sweet, juicy, or cooling in nature and give the body a balance from the accumulating heat of the season while nourishing us in this active time.

Finally, in the late summer and early autumn, the harvest of grains and heavy, dense vegetables brings foods that are more warming and building, to counter the mounting cold. The body uses these heavier foods to store up an extra layer of fat insulation for winter and to counteract the lightness and dryness of the climate. The season of storage is internal and external—we also store up roots and grains to last throughout the season, and then nuts, seeds, beans and—if we eat them—animal products like eggs, fats, and meats to supply what storage cannot. These foods are the most warming and heaviest and help insulate the body from the cold, dry, rough, and depleting nature of nature itself in the winter season. From here the cycle starts again, complete with a natural spring cleanse to clear out all the accumulations from the winter.

This is a beautiful yet simple system. The main challenge is that in our marketplace of abundance that lacks a strong connection to the natural environment, it is often difficult to know what to eat. The supermarkets have a harvest from the world at our fingertips in every season, and the choices change minimally with the seasons.

One way to stay connected with the natural seasonal harvest is to shop at a co-op that supports local farmers or at a nearby farmers' market. A resurgence in local and seasonal eating as a sustainable and environmentally friendly practice has made fresh, seasonal food more accessible to all—from farm-to-table restaurants to locally grown items highlighted in products, recipes, menus, and markets. Another option is to follow your tongue and choose foods with the appropriate tastes for each season: bitter, astringent and pungent in spring; sweet, bitter, and astringent in summer; and sweet, sour and salty in autumn and altering as necessary in winter.

Nature's Daily Cycle

The cycle of the seasons can offer information about what to eat, and the cycle of the day can tell us when to eat and when not to eat. The three doshas each predominate in a particular part of the day and night for approximately a four-hour period, and, if we understand this ebb and flow, we can make choices that will optimize our energy.

The sun sets in the evening, the temperature cools overnight, and by morning, moisture in the environment condenses. This is true in the mountains or the desert, in warm weather when you will see dew on the ground, or in cold weather

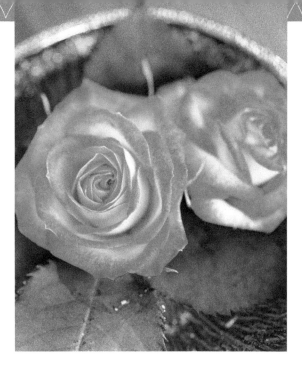

when you will see frost. The cool, moist, and heavy qualities that predominate at this time of the morning are like the kapha dosha (Mountain).

These qualities will have an effect on you. You might feel heavy if you wake late in the morning, and if you fall back to sleep, you feel even heavier then next time you wake. This feeling may be compounded if the weather also has cool, moist, and heavy qualities, as during a rainstorm; you might feel as if you need a crane to lift you out of bed. But by knowing the principle of opposites, you might counter this feeling with movement, exercise, a warm drink, a light and warming diet, or breath practices.

The peak of the sun at noon is also the peak of your digestive fire. The hot, light, and sharp qualities that are like pitta dosha (Fire) predominate at this time of day in both the external environment and your internal environment. It makes sense, then, to use this rising of fire to digest food. In fact, it is the ideal time for your biggest meal, because you have a better chance of complete digestion. It is also advisable to

Cycle of the Day

FIRE

— *day* —

Eat biggest meal

— *night* —

Sleep with
empty stomach

10 a.m./p.m.

2 a.m./p.m.

MOUNTAIN

— *day* —

Light meal and exercise
or movement

— *night* —

Light meal and
reduce stimulation
and activity

BREEZE

— *day* —

Reduce activity

— *night* —

Calm the body
for sound sleep

Sunrise 6 a.m.
Sunset 6 p.m.

use the principle of opposites to make good choices to cool the body. A vigorous training session for a marathon in the peak of the sun will definitely increase your fire. A gentle walk by a cool lake might be a better choice to keep the fire under control.

Vata dosha (Breeze) governs the transition times of the day, dusk and dawn, as they are related to change. The qualities of the Breeze, particularly mobility, increase at this time of day. The mind will become active and mobile, so these are good times for meditation. Too much physical mobility at this time of day may drain the reserves and leave you feeling tired. Ayurveda teaches us to eat our final meal early in the evening—so that we go to bed with a light stomach—and to enjoy a light meal, because the digestive fire is naturally lower at this time of day. In this transition time, the doshic cycle starts again.

Now it is important to slow down the body and mind during the second kapha time in preparation for a rejuvenating, sound sleep. Too much stimulation in the evening hours from television, computers, movies, or mental activity can impede this preparation. Calming practices of self-care, meditation, breathing practices, or relaxing yoga poses can help to nudge the body and mind into a restful state.

The second pitta time starts around 10 p.m., with an uprising of heat that can bring hunger again—we often recognize this energy as our "second wind." Once it starts, the fire or second wind does not subside until about 2 a.m. This surge of internal fire is intended to clean out any toxins in the body that have accumulated that day. If the belly is full, the fire will be digesting food, not cleaning the house. This self-maintenance will not be possible if you are not asleep between the hours of 10 p.m. and 2 a.m. It is therefore vital to eat a light meal, early in the evening, so that the belly can be empty before 10 p.m. Once the fire rises, it is difficult for sleep to happen (difficulty falling asleep at this time is likely due to a Fire imbalance). The second wind can be a useful time for creativity, work, or projects, but it comes at the expense of your sleep and therefore your health.

The final vata period of this cycle is in the early morning hours before and encompassing sunrise.

The mobility of the mind will predominate if sleep is not sound, creating insomnia. If this happens, use the practices for calming the nervous system in the daily self-care section of chapter 6 to relax and return to sleep. This is the time that yogis and other spiritual seekers traditionally choose to practice meditation, yoga, or chanting, to harness the energy of the mind and counter vata or Breeze imbalances.

During this time of the morning, the mobile quality stimulates the organs of elimination. It is advisable, therefore, to empty or clear the bladder, bowels, lungs, and skin upon rising, so that the body does not reabsorb the toxins eliminated through the self-maintenance of pitta overnight. Daily cleansing practices to clear the senses at this time are also recommended.

Waking around sunrise is advised for everyone, though each body-mind type has different sleep requirements that influence the ideal time. Mountain individuals require only five to six hours of sleep and may feel heavy and lethargic if they sleep more, so waking before sunrise is ideal. Fire individuals need about seven hours of sleep, so they can wake up at sunrise. Breeze individuals require the most sleep, so they can start the day an hour after sunrise.

Daily choices about how much to eat, what to eat, and when to eat, in addition to the basic dietary guidelines for each type, are the foundational building blocks of good health. The body also requires seasonal cleansing to remove toxins accumulated from our food, water, and air, as well as the excess doshas accumulated from the influence of the seasons, inappropriate lifestyle practices, and ignoring the intelligence of the body.

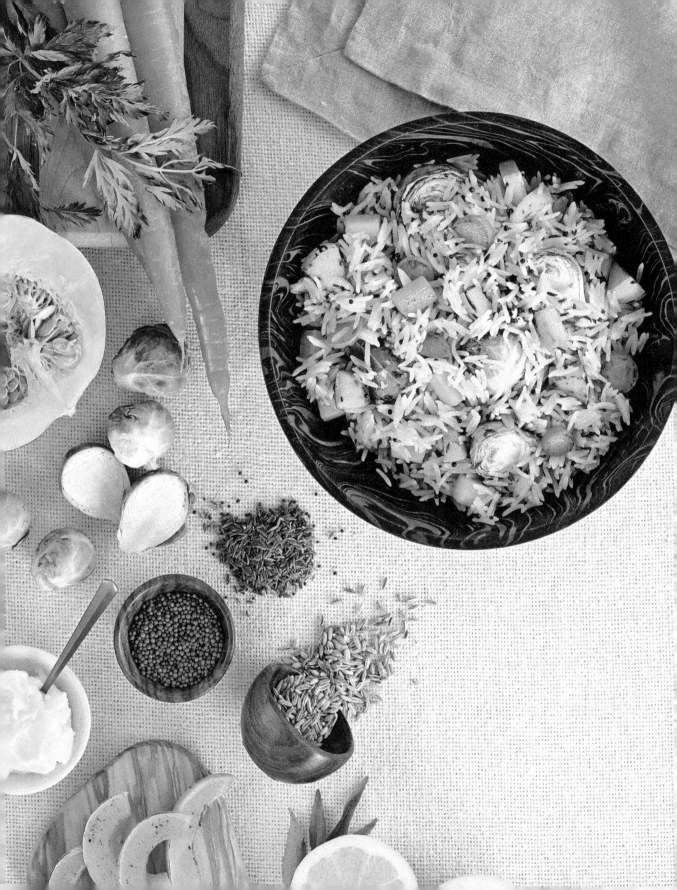

CHAPTER FOUR

Why Do We Need to Cleanse?

According to Ayurveda, a balanced digestive fire is one of the most important elements responsible for health in the body and, therefore, an imbalanced digestive fire is the first step in creation of disease. As we explored in the previous chapter, an imbalance of Breeze, Fire, or Mountain can lead to disruption of the normal digestive fire and formation of poor-quality tissues. This disruption can also lead to the production of a substance much like glue that can affect the proper functioning of the body. When this happens, cleansing is the only way to restore balance.

Understanding the Buildup of Toxins

Improperly processed or partially processed food creates a sticky substance that the body cannot use to build healthy tissues, and this substance is difficult to eliminate from the system. The substance is called *ama* in Ayurveda. Ama does not serve a physiological, healthy function in our bodies. On the contrary, it clogs channels, blocks the proper flow of nutrients, and prohibits waste removal, until it finally weakens the ability of your body to do its job. Physical symptoms such as stiff or achy joints, heaviness, lethargy, digestive discomfort, gas, bloating, acid reflux, bad breath, constipation, and diarrhea are all signs of accumulated ama.

Factors in accumulation of ama include poor dietary habits, imbalanced digestive fire, and imbalances or impairment of the natural function in the small intestine, the large intestines, the liver, the pancreas, or the lymphatic system. As we learned on page 39, we must also sleep with an empty stomach at the appropriate time of night, so that the body can accomplish the important job of self-cleaning. If wastes are excreted at the proper time of night but the organs of elimination are not cleaned or emptied in the morning, the body may reabsorb these toxins and ama. We must attend to all of these factors to prevent the accumulation of ama.

In addition to faulty eating practices and digestion creating ama, we are almost all exposed to chemical substances, cancer-causing agents, and toxins from the environment. These substances are also ama and are lipophilic, meaning that they attach to lipids, or fats, in the body, and the lymphatic system must detoxify and eliminate them. The lymphatic system is like our internal plumbing for waste removal, but it is also connected to our immune system, so that white blood cells can detoxify wastes and make them innocuous enough for removal through the blood stream and organs of elimination. The body does this job naturally, but many factors (as mentioned above) can impede this process and force the body to store these toxins instead of eliminating them.

The guiding intelligence of the body, knowing that ama will block normal functions of digestion, assimilation, and elimination, will try to store toxins and undigested sludge in a space outside of the digestive tract. Fat, or adipose tissue, is one main site of storage for toxins, to keep them out of circulation. Other spaces in the body that are weakened by trauma, injury, illness, and genetic inheritance, or inherently weak spots, can also become storage sites.

Once ama has been created and stored, we must use cleansing practices that lighten the body.

The classic texts of Ayurveda classify qualities, foods, and practices into two opposing categories. *Langhana*, or lightening, refers to qualities, foods, or actions that lighten the body or create a cleansing action. *Brahmana*, or building, is used to describe nourishing qualities, foods, and actions, employed when rejuvenation is needed. Lightening will remove stored wastes and can invigorate the body, but it will also weaken the body in the process, so building is required to return the tissues to fullness of strength. Each body-mind type is in need of these two actions, but some need more lightening and others more building due to their natural tendencies.

Reading the Tongue to Understand Imbalance

How do you know if you have ama? Very simply, your body tells you each day if the food from the previous day was digested properly. When you rise in the morning, look at your tongue in the mirror. If you see a coating on your tongue, you will know that you have not adequately digested your food. A thin, white coating that does not disguise the underlying color of your tongue is normal. Any other variation of coating is a sign that something needs to change.

Ayurveda and other Eastern systems, such as traditional Chinese medicine, consider the tongue a map of the body. Every feature of the tongue represents an aspect of the constitution or of imbalance. Any excess coating conveys an accumulation of waste products (ama) and a disruption in healthy processes of digestion, assimilation, or elimination. The tongue is the top end of a long, continuous tube that we call the digestive tract, and it acts as a mirror for the internal, or unseen, functioning of the system. The color of its coating can be a tool for understanding what imbalance is predominating in the body. Getting to know the signs of imbalance can lead you toward adjustments in diet and lifestyle to improve digestive function.

As a reminder from previous chapters, the three body-mind types each have a color or colors associated with imbalance. Accumulations anywhere in the body or in the waste products are white in color when influenced by a Mountain imbalance. Yellow or red are the colors associated with Fire imbalance. Dark brown or grayish discoloration is a sign of a Breeze imbalance. These colors are important to reading the body's messages that display themselves on the tongue every day.

For example, a thick yellow coating on the tongue with a bright red tongue base would indicate that the Fire is high. This might guide you, using the principle of langhana, to lighten the diet and, using the principle of opposites, to include more cooling foods with bitter and astringent tastes in your diet for the day. These two actions combined would help to reduce ama and cool the increased excess heat,

with any luck restoring balance. It may take one day or several days of these recommended actions, but the tongue will be the guide. Listen to the wisdom of the body and continue these actions until the yellow coating dissipates.

Alternately, if a thick white coating is predominant on the tongue and the base color is pale, a Mountain imbalance and ama are present. We often see this during a cold with congestion. In this case, lightening the diet or fasting to improve the strength of the digestive fire and ingesting strong pungent spices, along with astringent tastes, would burn up the accumulations of ama. A day of spicy, hot ginger and black pepper tea without the intake of food might be enough to clear up the ama—or several days of a light diet composed of pungent, bitter, and astringent foods may be adequate.

Ama is the fertile soil in which the seed of disease can grow. If we ignore the signs of imbalance, then toxins, ama, and excess doshas can accumulate and have an opportunity to spread to other parts of the body. According to Ayurveda, this accumulation marks the beginning stages, or precursors, of disease.

The Six Stages of Disease

Imbalance follows a logical progression in the body to the point at which disease manifests, and Ayurveda reveals the steps and symptoms along this journey. Each dosha has a natural site—its homesite—in the digestive tract, where it functions healthfully. Accumulation happens here first, bringing with it minor symptoms of imbalance. It then becomes aggravated in the second stage of dis-ease, bringing stronger imbalances. If allowed to continue in its progression, the dosha will enter the third stage: an overflow from the digestive tract

WHAT IS YOUR TONGUE SAYING?

- Color of the tongue body: pink or dark/ Breeze; bright red/Fire; or pale/Mountain

- Dark or brownish coating: ama with Breeze imbalance

- Yellow coating: ama with Fire imbalance

- Thick, white coating: ama with Mountain imbalance

into other sites in the body, and will also create imbalance there.

In the fourth stage of dis-ease (spreading), the accumulated doshas and ama move through the body's channels of circulation and look for a weak site—called *khavaigunya*—in various tissues and organs to make their home. There, they begin to alter the normal qualities of those tissues. In the fifth stage of dis-ease, (relocation), the dosha becomes more rooted in its new home and its qualities become more defined and pronounced as signs and symptoms of illness. Finally in the sixth stage (manifestation), the dosha has not only invaded one place, but has also aggravated surrounding organs and tissues, resulting in a substantial disease complete with symptoms and complications.

> *"Just as rasa nourishes its*
> *fellow tissues, ama is the juice*
> *that nourishes disease."*

—**Dr. Robert Svoboda, Bachelor of Ayurvedic Medicine and Surgery**

Why wait until disease manifests to listen to the body? Ayurveda gives us the tools to recognize imbalance and stop it before it progresses into disease. One weakness of our modern system of medicine is that we cannot spot most diseases in the precursor stages and, therefore, prevention is limited. What we often call "early detection" is when a disease is already in the fourth or fifth stage. True early detection is when we can identify a disorder in the first or second stage of disease, and disease prevention is when we can prevent progression into further, more serious stages and even guide those stages backward.

Cleansing Basics

Just as there is no single diet appropriate for everyone, no one cleanse is right for everyone. The range of cleanses on the market today is wide and varied. One cleanse may have its participants drinking only liquids for forty days while another requires consumption of only animal proteins and vegetables for a week. There are three-day cleanses for the weekend warrior and three-week intensives that require incredible amounts of discipline to complete. Each type of cleanse is appropriate for someone, but without the framework of Ayurveda it can be difficult to understand which one is right for you.

Your current imbalance is the main factor to consider when determining which type of cleanse to undertake. Evaluating your imbalance each time you decide to cleanse is important, because the relative state of balance or imbalance in our bodies is constantly changing with our geography, the climate, and the season, as well as our diet, lifestyle, and stage of life. If you do not have a single predominant imbalance, choose a cleanse based on your constitution with a mindful consideration to the season in which you are cleansing. A cleanse that is right for your type is crucial if you are looking to create better health without more imbalance.

When to Cleanse

Ayurveda specifies the junctions between seasons as the ideal time for cleansing, to clear out any accumulation before it can cause problems in the body. With the exception of the extremes of hot and cold in your climate (see sidebar on page 46), any season is permissible. Cleansing one to three times per year is good maintenance, and this is especially true around the season that is most like your predominant type. For example, it is a good idea for everyone to cleanse at the beginning or end of summer, to clear out accumulated heat in the body before it creates a problem. This is especially important for Fire types, because that additional heat on top of their naturally strong fire will create problems if it is held in the body too long. Mountain types have a greater need to clear out the heavy, moist accumulations in the spring, and Breeze types have a stronger need to counter the cold and dry of fall before the winter arrives.

Cleansing Guidelines for the Breeze

In general, cleansing is most challenging for a Breeze type because cleanses are inherently lightening and the qualities of Breeze are light already. The challenge is to employ sufficient grounding techniques to ensure that the Breeze type will not get more aggravated by cleansing. A **grounding cleanse**, which incorporates warm, well-cooked foods that are easy to digest, is perfect for Breeze individuals or those with a Breeze imbalance. This gives their digestive system a break from more-complicated foods and preserves their delicate digestive fire. A fast, or a diet consisting of only liquid foods such as fresh vegetable juice, herbal teas, and sometimes, exclusively water, is too lightening for the Breeze individual. A diet of only raw foods is too cold and difficult for them to digest, plus the large amount of fiber in those raw foods can be rough and abrasive to their sensitive and often dry colons. Breeze individuals might feel unbearably cold, ungrounded, or anxious from those types of cleanses, responses that lead to more imbalance than health.

Too much change, too quickly in diet and lifestyle, can deplete immunity in Breeze types. They are already light, cold, and sensitive by nature, and need a gentle change. Along with incorporating warming foods, it is essential for the Breeze individual to rest more and engage in grounding practices like gentle yoga, warming breath practices, meditation, and warm oil massage during a cleanse, to enable them to complete the process in a safe, supported way. Adequate time away from the stresses of life is also important to the success of any cleanse, as the Breeze imbalance is directly related to the function of the nervous system.

In any season, a short cleanse or mono diet—a simplifying of the diet by eating one type of food—will serve these individuals, but it is especially important to cleanse in the fall before the weather gets too cold. Proper time and focus on rejuvenation is essential, particularly in the fall, so that the tissues and digestive fire have time to rebuild and move into winter with strength. Chapter 8 has more information to help the Breeze address their specific needs.

Cleansing Guidelines for the Mountain

Mountain types need cleansing that reduces the bulk of their body while still keeping the digestive fire burning strong. They have larger stores of muscle and fat, creating a thicker layer of insulation than the other types have, so although all cleanses tend to be a bit lightening, Mountains need an especially **lightening cleanse** to reduce the bulk of the body. In addition, the stable nature of these individuals enables them to remain grounded and maintain their strength during a dramatic shift in diet. Therefore, a cleanse involving fasting on water or vegetable juice could be acceptable for them in certain conditions, as this forces their bodies to burn accumulated fat stores for energy, greatly reducing the amount of body mass.

But the Mountain type still needs enough heat or fire to keep everything moving. Too much cold from consuming only liquids may cause their digestive system to slow down, dramatically impairing the body's ability to remove wastes and toxins. A lightening cleanse with bitter, astringent, and pungent foods may be more effective than a fast alone. These foods stimulate catabolic activity, the breakdown and removal of old cells and accumulations, while keeping the digestive fire burning strong. In addition, vigorous exercise, exposure to the sun, dry sauna, or other forms of heat that induce sweating will greatly increase the lightening aspects of a cleanse.

Springtime cleansing is most important for the Mountain individual or those with a Mountain imbalance. The accumulated stores from winter need to be eliminated early in the spring or else the liquefying process that kapha undergoes as the weather warms will create uncomfortable symptoms, including sinus congestion, lung congestion, runny nose, itchy eyes, sneezing, headaches in the frontal area around the sinuses, heaviness, lethargy, weight gain, and water retention. These individuals can undergo a long and rigorous cleansing process in any season, but it is particularly helpful in the spring. Chapter 7 has more specific information to help the Mountain plan an appropriate cleanse.

Cleansing Guidelines for the Fire

The Fire types need a **cooling cleanse**, with enough food to keep their strong digestive fire satisfied. A Fire's robust appetite must be satiated by food regularly or the excess heat that builds up creates an imbalance. Fasting or eating too little food could create an internal inferno and disrupt the nervous system. The physical and emotional fire that could potentially build up may counter any other health benefits from a cleanse. Raw foods combined with fresh juice may be appropriate in a hot season or climate, but a mono diet of easily digested foods would be better in a cool season or climate.

Cooling practices that are also calming in nature are ideal to include in a cleanse for this type. Gentle and cooling yoga poses and breath work, easy, noncompetitive exercise in or near water, and massage with cooling oils are all good practices to

CONTRAINDICATIONS FOR CLEANSING

Winter in many regions is a season for storage and insulation, and our bodies naturally bulk up in the cooling fall season to insulate against the cold of winter. Cleansing in the winter in a cold climate is not ideal, because the body requires heavy, oily, and warming foods to counter the cold, dry, rough, and depleting qualities present in the season. Classic Ayurvedic textbooks advise traditional cleansing (we will explore the difference between this and modern cleansing) in this season only when it is a health emergency and only if one can avoid the effects of cold during the process. The texts recommend avoiding elimination therapies in the extremes of your climate—both the peak of heat in the summer and during the winter's extreme cold. Cleansing is also not appropriate for pregnant women, nursing mothers, young children, women during their menses, or anyone in a weakened condition from illness or trauma.

incorporate into a cleanse. In addition, time away from the world of stimulation and activity gives the mind a well-needed rest.

Heat can easily accumulate in cool seasons, when the external cold encourages the body to hold heat internally, and also in hot seasons, when the influence of the external heat has a powerful effect despite adequate self-care. So cleansing at the beginning or end of the warm summer season—or both—is beneficial for the Fire types or those with a Fire imbalance. Chapter 8 has more specific information to help the Fire individual determine the unique combination of elements to incorporate into a cleanse.

Cleansing with the Cycle of the Seasons

A healthy individual with no regular tongue coating and only occasional symptoms of imbalance could use three different cleanses seasonally to maintain health. A grounding cleanse will gently clear the body of accumulations in the fall while maintaining immunity, warmth, and strength for the coming winter. A lightening cleanse is great for spring when the extra insulation from winter needs to be lifted. A cooling cleanse is ideal to counter the heat of summer. This framework of understanding from Ayurvedic wisdom can help make sense of the enormous amount of conflicting information available today about diet, nutrition, and cleansing. Each individual cleanse or style of eating is good for someone, but knowing which one will work for you takes a little deeper knowledge of yourself.

The Categories of Cleansing

Traditional Ayurvedic cleansing is a practice of lightening the body, so that it can eliminate internal accumulations of toxins from the environment, ama from undigested foods, and excess doshas. This systematic cleansing and rejuvenation is called *panchakarma*. Cleansing steps include cleaning or clearing the digestive tract by strengthening the digestive fire and reducing ama, then oleating, or softening with oil applications, the body internally and externally so that it can remove the excess doshas and toxins from deeper storage through elimination therapies (see chapter 9 for more details). Most cleansing practices or packages available on the market either (a) lighten the body by reducing bulk in the diet; or (b) clear and clean the digestive tract, which is the first, but not the only step of traditional Ayurvedic cleansing. Most of these modern cleanses, however, do not address the accumulation of doshas.

Since all of these processes come under the term *cleansing*, it is important to differentiate between discrete categories. The first cleansing category involves processes that assist the body in its natural daily cleansing. These include sound sleep at the appropriate time of night, and potentially a massage, healing therapy, or daily practice (like the simple daily routine of cleansing, *dinacharya*, on page 57) that moves the lymphatic system or opens the channels, as well as appropriate diet for your type and season, to pacify the doshas and prevent further production of ama. We will call these **daily cleansing** practices.

The second category relates to lightening practices, which for our purposes have three subcategories. The first is **dietary cleansing** and is defined as changing the diet to include lighter food choices. Many modern cleanses fall under this category. Eating a vegetarian or vegan diet could be a simple example for those in the practice of eating meat, dairy, or other animal products. For someone accustomed to a vegan or vegetarian diet, dietary cleansing could happen by choosing a mono diet of exclusively fruit, exclusively vegetables, or kitchari

(the main mono diet used in Ayurveda). These dietary cleansing practices may or may not clear and clean the digestive tract.

We will refer to those lightening practices that improve the digestive fire and burn up ama as **digestive cleansing**. Examples of this include a fast or a mono diet (but only if it is appropriate for your imbalance and accomplishes those two aims). For example, a fast from food while consuming only strongly heating herbal teas would be an appropriate digestive cleanse for a Mountain. But a fast of only cold, moist fruit or vegetable juices could dampen the dull digestive fire of a Mountain and create more ama, even though this diet is lightening in nature; this would be considered a dietary cleanse, but not a digestive cleanse.

In an Ayurvedic mono diet of kitchari (see page 60), the whole digestive system gets a break from more complex or difficult-to-digest foods while consumption of herbal teas balances the digestive fire to address ama. The first stage of panchakarma, translated as *ama burning*, is another example of digestive cleansing during which an Ayurvedic practitioner would recommend specific dietary and herbal changes to clear up ama (see chapter 9).

The final category relates to lightening practices that help remove excess doshas and toxins from storage and is specific to Ayurveda. This includes the oleation and elimination phases of panchakarma. This is different from pacifying the doshas. In daily life, appropriate diet and lifestyle practices can calm any excessive doshas and reduce symptoms of imbalance, but at some point (after pacifying), it is advisable to remove the old accumulations from storage. This is equivalent to pulling up the roots of dis-ease as opposed to just trimming the plants that sprout from imbalance. All the recommendations from the classic Ayurvedic texts refer to this type of cleansing, which we will call **eliminatory cleansing**, which refers to the use of elimination therapies of panchakarma (see chapter 9).

Another difference between traditional Ayurvedic cleansing and modern cleansing is the focus on preliminary practices before cleansing and rejuvenation practices after cleansing. Ayurveda would recommend a cleanse only after appropriate dietary and lifestyle habits have been established, so that the doshas will be pacified or calmed. A cleanse would also be followed by a period of rejuvenation in which proper diet and self-care practices would have the utmost importance, to restore strength to the body before returning to a "normal" daily routine and diet. These preliminary practices and rejuvenating steps are just as important as the cleansing time itself; otherwise, the health of the body may be diminished instead of improved. All too often cleansing ends abruptly without a plan for reintegrating into one's normal diet and routine. Inappropriate diet or practices at this time when the body is vulnerable can potentially be damaging.

Part II of this book incorporates these preparation and rejuvenation practices, as well as daily cleansing, dietary cleansing, and digestive cleansing practices, into a 31-day protocol for better health. Each one of us is unique and we need to determine which type of cleanse and how much lightening is appropriate for our imbalance, constitution, or both. By applying the knowledge of Ayurveda presented in Part I of this book, we can move on to choosing a cleanse that lightens in just the right amount while maintaining or regaining balance.

HOW MUCH WATER SHOULD I CONSUME EACH DAY?

Ayurvedic texts provide only simple guidelines for water intake based on one's constitution. From my personal experience, eight glasses of water is a good general guideline, but again, each body is unique.

Breeze individuals need the most water to counter their dry tendency (eight 10-ounce glasses: 80 ounces or 2.4 liters daily). Fire individuals will have a moderate need for water (seven glasses: 70 ounces or 2 liters daily). Mountain individuals typically need less water (six glasses: 60 ounces or 1.8 liters daily). In general, our own natural intelligence can guide how much water we drink, if we truly pay attention to our thirst—although many people mistake the need for water as hunger. Our bodies will naturally need more water if we are in warm, dry climates or environments, or if we are exercising and sweating regularly.

If you consume coffee, black or green tea, other caffeinated beverages, or alcohol, which dehydrate the body, you may need to consume extra water to compensate. One additional ounce of water per ounce of caffeinated or alcoholic beverage is a good estimate. A person who drinks a 12-ounce (0.35 liter) cup of coffee in the morning and two 8-ounce glasses (0.5 liter) of wine in the evening should drink an additional 28 ounces (0.8 liter) of water in a day.

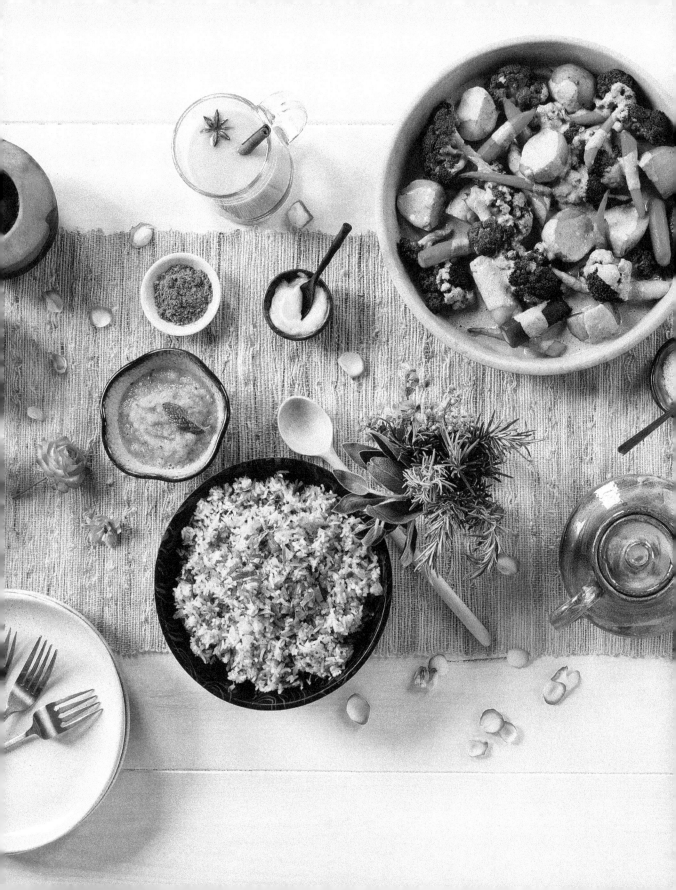

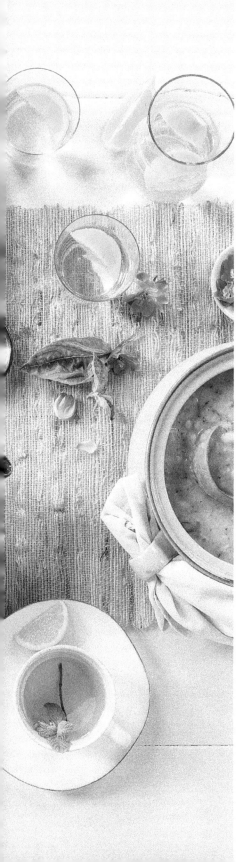

PART 2

Cleansing for Your Body-Mind Type

The recipes, lifestyle changes, and self-care practices from this book combine to prepare the body, help bring about a gentle Ayurvedic cleanse, and safely transition back to daily living. These practices make up a 31-day protocol that is explained in chapter 5, but they can always be used for everyday living. After a cleanse, slowly move back to your normal diet and schedule while maintaining the practices you find create the most balance.

If you engage in seasonal cleansing regularly, you may notice that the differences between your "normal" and "cleansing" routines lessen over time. When that happens, you will be ready to engage in more traditional Ayurvedic cleansing (see chapter 9). At that point, the 31-day protocol, which balances the doshas and removes ama and toxins from the digestive tract, will become the preliminary practices to prepare you for eliminatory cleansing that removes deeply rooted excess doshas.

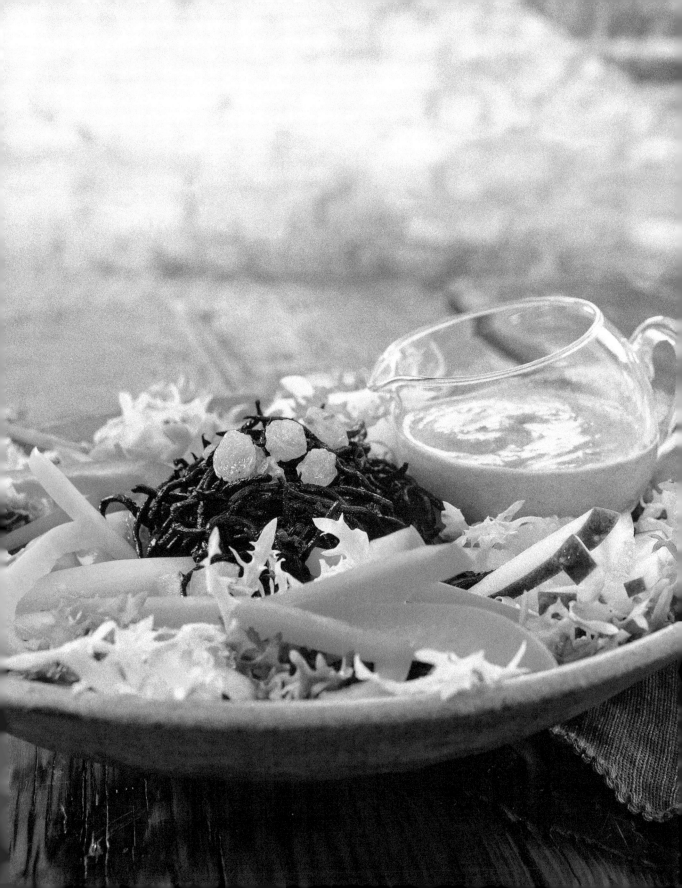

CHAPTER FIVE

Simple Eating for Everyone

This chapter provides a 31-day protocol that is simple, gentle, and safe for almost everyone. It is designed to create more awareness about food choices and help you to listen to the wisdom of your own body. However, if you have specific health concerns, please consult your physician or health care practitioner to determine whether this diet and the cleanses in this book are right for you.

The first three weeks of the protocol incorporate daily cleansing practices and are the same for everyone, with minimal changes to the diet. The focus, instead, is applying the knowledge of Ayurveda to determine how much to eat, where to eat, and when to eat. These three weeks will give you the foundations for lifelong healthy eating practices.

The fourth week includes dietary cleansing practices that you will choose specifically for your imbalance (or constitution, if there is no predominant imbalance). It will lay out a plan complete with diet and lifestyle recommendations for creating balance. The final three days are the digestive cleansing days, with a limited diet and limited activity. The final segment of this chapter, Transition Time, will also give you suggestions for easing out of the cleanse in a safe and timely manner.

Week 1

— finding balance with portion size —

The first week requires no change to your diet, but instead focuses on discovering the right amount of food for each meal. To start, find a bowl that fits perfectly in your two hands and holds the same amount as your two hands cupped together. Fill the bowl only two-thirds full, as the stomach should ideally be one-third full of solid food, one-third full of liquid foods, and one-third with space. Use this bowl when you are eating at home, so that you have a good visual estimate of the proper amount of food.

When the stomach reaches its ideal capacity, as just described, the body creates a signal: a small burp or uprising energy from your stomach. It might be a silent, bubble-like sensation or a fully audible belch. During meals, give special attention to listening for your burp. It may surprise you to see how early the burp arrives. Once it happens, notice if you feel content or satiated with this amount of food. If not, count the number of bites it takes after the burp to find contentment.

This is your only practice for the week, so try to give it your full attention at every meal. As the week progresses, notice any changes to your awareness. Are you able to recognize the burp at each meal or do you still miss it? Can you predict when the burp will arrive, based on the amount of food you consumed? Are you closer to contentment when it arrives? If the answer is no, observe yourself at meals. Is anything distracting you— conversations, work, television, or something else?

Week 2

— mindful eating: what are you feeding yourself? —

This week, you will shift your attention to the manner and setting in which you eat, as well as the overall quality of the food you consume. You will begin to eliminate stimulating foods from your diet and start consuming more calming foods. The question to ask is, "What am I feeding myself?" The answer may be more complex than you think.

Once you have knowledge of Ayurveda, it is easy to see that the twenty qualities are in and around us at every moment. Our emotions, thoughts, sensory perceptions, conversations, environment, food, and the seasons all affect us. At mealtimes, other qualities are "ingested" along with our food. The question to ask is, "Can I also 'digest' these qualities?" When it comes to emotions, those such as grief, sadness, anger, or fear can completely stamp out the digestive fire. For this reason Ayurveda recommends eating only when emotions are calm and stable.

On a more subtle level, this concept is true for all of the components present during a meal. A busy, loud, and stimulating environment may affect the nervous system and decrease the strength of the digestive fire. An uncomfortably hot, moist setting or season can inflame or impair the appetite. A stimulating conversation, television program, or book can divert energy away from the belly to the mind, slowing digestion. We must have enough power to digest our food as well as the qualities we are "feeding" ourselves during each meal.

In Ayurveda, three categories classify the basic energetics, the action or essence predominant in a substance or activity, of the mind, food, and activities—calming, stimulating, or dulling. Foods that are calming in nature (*sattvic*, or the natural state of the mind) create a sense of stillness, peace, clarity, purity, and contentment. Foods that are stimulating in nature (*rajasic*) create movement and heat, bringing with them cravings, irritations, and desire for more stimulation. Dulling foods (*tamasic*) create inertia of body and mind with heavy, cloudy, and lethargic sensations.

The qualities of foods, environment, and mind affect digestion. For example, a quiet, peaceful environment for meals can create a calm state of mind; a violent television program or emotions of anger can create a heated, stimulated state of mind; and news of a tragic event can trigger a heavy, dull state of mind. Eating calming foods in a calming setting with calm emotions will have the result of a calm body and mind: This is the goal.

Look at the lists that follow and notice whether the foods you consume regularly are calming, stimulating, or dulling. This week, start to eliminate the stimulating and dulling foods, so that by the end of it you are eating mostly calming foods. Eliminate alcohol, coffee, caffeinated foods or beverages, carbonated drinks, processed white sugar and flour, packaged, canned, and fast foods, deep-fried foods, and red meat for the remainder of the month. Try to eat freshly prepared foods whenever possible, particularly those you make yourself.

Notice the environment in which you eat regularly. What other qualities are you feeding yourself? Start to shift your habits by eating in a quiet and calm environment, avoiding television, work, computers, or reading, and limiting conversations. Take time to focus on the process of digestion and your enjoyment of the tastes, textures, colors, and aromas of your food. Use all your senses, and chew slowly and thoroughly. Continue to listen for your burp and be aware of contentment when it arises.

Energetics of Food

Calming foods are naturally sweet and building in nature. They include the following:

- fresh fruits and vegetables (except heating ones)

- whole grains, particularly rice, wheat, quinoa, and oats

- beans (in moderation), especially mung, aduki, or soy/tofu

- raw soaked nuts and seeds of almonds, sesame seeds, cashews, and coconut

- raw and/or organic dairy products from cows or goats that have been treated well, especially milk, ghee, soft cheese, or homemade yogurt

- natural sweeteners, such as raw sugar, raw honey, maple syrup, and jaggery

- moderate amounts of sweet spices such as ginger, cardamom, cinnamon, fennel, cumin, coriander, and saffron

- garden herbs, such as mint, basil, cilantro, and tulsi

- food prepared with love and awareness

Stimulating foods are highly seasoned, heating in nature, and create movement. They include:

- coffee, caffeinated beverages, and chocolate

- carbonated drinks

- heating and sour fruits, such as sour oranges, guava, tamarind, and pineapple

- heating vegetables, such as radishes, eggplant, garlic, peppers, and onions

- millet and corn

- nuts (except almonds, cashews, coconut, peanuts, or rancid nuts)

- dairy products that are sour, such as sour cream or buttermilk

- seafood and chicken

- heating spices such as black pepper, chili pepper, paprika, and curry

- heating garden herbs, such as rosemary, thyme, oregano, and chives

- refined, artificial, or highly processed sweeteners

Dulling foods are heavy, lacking prana (energy), stale, partially cooked, overcooked, fruits that are overripe or under ripe, and processed sweets or overly processed foods in general. They include:

- alcohol

- garlic, onions, and mushrooms

- processed, refined, and bleached flour of grains

- wheat

- urad dal (legume)

- peanuts and rancid nuts

- hard cheese and highly processed dairy products

- red meats

- nutmeg and jalepeño

- molasses and highly-processed stevia

- canned, frozen, or highly processed foods

Note: Mountain individuals need some stimulating foods to create internal heat and movement, and Breeze individuals can also tolerate a small amount. Unless living a life of seclusion or meditation and contemplation, the Fire and Breeze types usually require some amount of heavy and dulling foods to build strength and keep them heavy enough to do their work in the world and sleep soundly.

Week 3
— attuning to the cycle of the day —

Now you will shift your attention to eating at the proper times of day, drinking a proper amount of water for your type at appropriate times, and developing rituals for mealtimes, mornings, and evenings. This will bring you stability, ensure better digestion and elimination, and establish basic self-care practices you will expand in week 4.

Review the cycle of the day from chapter 4 (pages 37 to 39) and notice ways you can adjust your schedule to accommodate these recommendations. Start with meals: Eat your largest or heaviest meal at noon, eat lighter meals in the morning and evening, and eat at established and regular times every day. Find ways to make your meals feel like a sacred ritual: Light a candle, express gratitude for the food, take a few deep breaths and calm yourself before eating, or have a special cup of tea before or after meals. Continue to use all the practices from weeks 1 and 2 at every meal.

Review the section on water intake (page 49) and determine the proper amount you need. Make a plan to incorporate water breaks in the day so that you consume an adequate amount without impeding digestion: Drink one hour before or two hours after a meal (see the daily schedule in chapters 6 to 8 for a sample plan). Start with a large glass of warm water upon rising and then carry a glass or stainless steel water bottle with you throughout the day, so that you can drink when you are thirsty. Water is essential for the cleansing process, as it carries wastes from the body through urine and sweat, stimulates peristaltic movement to eliminate the bowels, and hydrates the lymphatic system, which is the body's plumbing.

Create a basic morning and evening routine for simple self-care, with regular times for sleeping and waking. Take ten minutes in the morning and evening for self-care practices. In the morning, take time to clean each of the senses—eyes, ears, nose, and tongue—in addition to eliminating wastes (bowels and bladder). In the evening, take a warm bath, practice deep belly breaths (see page 75), or sit in stillness before bedtime. The simple daily routine below for morning is part of a daily routine of cleansing practices, or *dinacharya*, that is recommended in week 4, and we will add more specific morning and evening self-care recommendations for your type in chapters 6 to 8.

Simple Daily Routine for Morning

- Drink warm water.

- Eliminate waste from the bowels and bladder.

- Observe the tongue and coating, then swish one teaspoon of sesame oil in the mouth for five to ten minutes and spit it out; brush teeth and scrape the tongue (with a tongue scraper or edge of a spoon).

- Splash the eyes with cool water—or if they are red or irritated, spritz with rose water.

- Use a neti pot to clear the sinuses of excess mucus or use a few drops of sesame oil in each nostril if you have no congestion.

- Place one or two drops of sesame oil in each ear and massage with a fingertip.

Week 4
— dietary cleanse for your type —

The fourth week incorporates a dietary cleanse by eating a vegetarian diet that eliminates heavier food choices like cheese, bread, and pasta. For this week, you will choose one cleanse—grounding, lightening, or cooling—and follow the recommended recipes and lifestyle practices for it (see chapters 6 to 8). Choose the right cleanse for you based on your **current predominant imbalance** (use the Imbalance Checklist from the appendix to determine your imbalance; see page 139.) Choose the grounding cleanse for a Breeze imbalance, the cooling cleanse for a Fire imbalance, and the lightening cleanse for a Mountain imbalance. If you have more than one predominant imbalance, see the Cleansing Table (page 140) to decide which cleanse is right for you. If you have no predominant imbalance, choose a cleanse based on your constitution with mindful consideration of the season (see page 141).

Once you choose your cleanse, read through the appropriate chapter to make sure that it feels right for you. Each dietary cleansing chapter has recipes specific to one body-mind type or season, but every recipe also has variations for the other body-mind types. For example, you can modify any of the recipes in the lightening cleanse for the Fire type. If you have a predominant Mountain imbalance but know that you cannot handle strong heating spices because of your Fire constitution, use the lightening cleanse with the Fire modifications. This will give you the information you need to adjust your cleanse and make it fitting for you.

Final Cleansing Days

The final three days following week 4 incorporate digestive cleansing practices. You will eat **only foods from the Basic Cleansing Staples section on page 60** and drink **only warm water or warm herbal teas** from the cleanse you chose in week 4. This will give the digestive system a break and strengthen the digestive fire enough to burn up ama and toxins in the digestive tract. Choose only the following:

- whole and freshly cooked foods

- warm, simple foods

- warm or room-temperature drinks

It is also a time to rest and give the body and mind a break from activity. Eliminate all exercise and yoga (except Bed Yoga; see below); choose gentle breathing practices and meditation from the self-care section of chapter 6 (see page 75); take a break from all electronics and mental stimulation, and rest as much as possible. Avoid the following:

- exercise, vigorous breathing practices, or strenuous activities

- a busy schedule, including excessive activities or movement

- mental work or stimulation from computers, cell phones, television, and other electronic devices

Continue all other daily self-care practices for your type, including oil massage or raw silk massage.

The last three days of digestive cleansing involve an Ayurvedic mono diet of foods from the basic staples. If digestion is a challenge for you, to simplify even further, you can limit what you eat to kitchari. The most important part of these three days is eating foods that are easy to digest, so listen to your body and make changes if you are having digestive discomforts. As the body eliminates toxins, you may experience other bodily discomforts, such as aches and pains, headaches, nausea, or excessive heaviness or feeling of exhaustion; these cleansing reactions are natural and will pass. You should feel a lightness in the body by the end of the 31-day protocol.

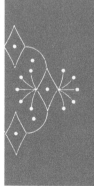

BED YOGA

During my panchakarma in India, I was advised to take complete rest—no activity or exercise, including yoga. But spending five weeks with little movement was challenging, so we compromised by doing only the stretches we could do gently and comfortably in bed—reclining, supported, and relaxing poses for the most part, with an occasional twist, arm stretch, or a seated forward fold. This turned out to be my favorite yoga for a long time. Try this during your cleanse, but if it is difficult to do in bed, it is probably too much for the final days of digestive cleansing.

Transition Time

After the final cleansing days, it is time to return slowly to your normal routine. Ending your cleansing time by jumping quickly back to many stimulating or dulling foods, heavy foods, or foods inappropriate for your type or the season could be detrimental to your health. Start by returning for a few days to the dietary cleanse you used in week 4 and choose mostly warm, cooked foods.

Introduce some heavier, more nourishing foods such as mushroom or bone broth (if you eat meat) at the end of the first week. Include raw foods only if appropriate for your type and the season, but be attentive to how your body feels with each new food you add. Notice if digestion feels easy or disturbed, so that you can continue to make food your medicine. Also, pay attention to your tongue coating every day and see if you can use your body's wisdom to help you make mindful food choices.

In the first week following your cleanse, keep it simple—both in diet and in activity. Try not to jump full force into everything. Start with gentle or moderate exercise and yoga, and for Mountain types, move back to vigorous exercise only when you are feeling your usual strength. Try to maintain the daily self-care practices you find helpful and make routines for health and balance a mainstay in your life. Leave out the need for perfection (Fire types, especially) and try to make your daily routine feel supportive and full of ease.

In the second week after the cleanse, reincorporate foods such as meat if you choose to consume it, but remember that it is a concentrated food and keep portions small. You can indulge a little more with richer foods, but notice the effect that these choices have on your body, energy, mind, and emotions. As you cleanse and become more balanced, the foods you once enjoyed may or may not be right for you. Leave some flexibility in your mind for the idea that certain food choices will no longer work for you. This is a sign of progress—that the practices of awareness about food and the cleanse have made a permanent change and you may experience a "new normal."

Finally, use some or all of the awareness practices from the protocol in everyday living. Use the practices of "simple eating" to remind yourself to listen to your own wisdom. Come back periodically to the simple diet plans from week 4 and the basic staples for each season or when your food choices have gone astray—even if you do not have time for the final cleansing days. This happens to all of us when we are busy, stressed, challenged emotionally, or out of our natural routine or environment. Nothing feels better to me after a week of travel than simple, home-cooked meals like kitchari (see pages 60 to 61). I actually crave it!

MODIFICATIONS OF THE CLEANSE

When the basic practices from the 31-day protocol become part of your everyday life, consider modifying the protocol to make the digestive cleansing section longer. Combine all of the practices from the first four weeks into one or two weeks so the digestive cleansing phase is seven to ten days instead of three. Once you have accomplished this without cleansing reactions, listed to the left, you are ready for the deeper cleansing practices in chapter 11 and should consult an Ayurvedic physician or practitioner for guidance.

Basic Cleansing Staple Recipes

From an Ayurvedic perspective, the simpler the diet, the better the cleansing effect. In traditional Ayurvedic cleanses, the following staples are the only foods consumed for several weeks or months. In fact, Ayurvedic practitioners often advise us to eat bland foods during panchakarma to avoid overstimulating the senses. The staples consist of mostly calming foods that are easy to digest and well cooked to give the digestive system a break.

You can use these recipes at any time during your 31-day protocol. They are especially good during the fourth week, when you can incorporate them into any of the cleanses. These staples are the exclusive diet for the final three days of the Ayurvedic mono diet, or digestive cleansing days. As you progress over time with your seasonal cleansing, consider using less variety in the diet and using mostly staples for the duration of the 31 days.

KITCHARI INGREDIENTS, EXPLAINED

Basmati rice is a brown or white aromatic whole grain. After harvesting, only the hull is removed, so it retains all of its natural nutrients, bran, and fiber. White basmati rice is milled a second time to remove the bran, reducing its nutritional content but making it easier to digest. The brown version has a heartier, nuttier taste, but since it is slightly harder to digest, it can be used for kitchari only when the digestive fire is strong and balanced.

Mung beans (Vigna radiata) have three varieties and many natural colors. The most common is green, and it is sold whole, or intact; split (appearing green); or split with the skins removed (appearing pale yellow).

The **split yellow mung** is so soft that it can easily turn to a smooth soup when cooked. In kitchari, this bean may lose its shape and become homogenously mashed with the rice. This is the best bean for those who have a delicate digestive tract, for deep cleansing, or for rejuvenation when the digestive fire is weak.

Split green mung beans have more fiber due to their skins, and require more water to cook thoroughly. When cooked with rice, they maintain their shape. I have heard that the added fiber is better for Breeze digestion or those with a history of constipation. To me, it feels slightly rough. If you feel this roughness, add more ghee and spices.

The **whole green mung bean** looks like a small, perfectly round green pearl. It is more dense and solid than both split beans, but faster to cook and easier to digest than other legumes like pinto or black beans. It is perfect to use in soups, as the added water content will soften the bean thoroughly.

You can use any of these beans in kitchari—and you can choose the type of grain according to the needs of each person eating it.

Kitchari

Kitchari is a nourishing dish made with equal parts mung beans and basmati rice often recommended as the ideal food in Ayurvedic cleansing and rejuvenation. The mung bean is the smallest, lightest, easiest bean to digest, and combined with basmati rice, it makes a complete protein that is easy to digest. It is mildly spiced to support healthy digestion, so more bodily energy can be devoted to the cleansing process. The ingredients in kitchari are also calming in nature, so the end result is a body and mind that are still, stable, and free of cravings. This combination is not too heating or cooling in nature; it is tri-doshic, or equally balanced.

Changing the amount of water in the recipe varies the consistency from a firm grain to porridge to a soup. This recipe uses white basmati, split yellow mung, and a tri-doshic spice mix. Variations appear for each type, but you can also adjust the recipe to your liking.

YIELD • FOUR 1-CUP (200 G) SERVINGS (UP TO SIX SERVINGS WHEN MADE INTO SOUP)

3–4 cups (705–946 ml) water

½ cup (95 g) white basmati rice

½ cup (92 g) split yellow mung beans

¼ cup (25 g) chopped asparagus

¼ cup (33 g) chopped carrots

¼ cup (25 g) chopped cauliflower

¼ cup (30 g) chopped yellow squash

1 tablespoon ghee (7 g) or coconut oil, if you prefer a vegan option

1 tablespoon (7 g) Simple spice mix (see page 86)

1 teaspoon salt (7 g)

splash of apple cider vinegar or a squeeze of lemon

Serve with:

1 sliced lemon or lime

¼ cup (4 g) chopped cilantro

salt

chutney (see page 85)

One-pot cooking method: Place the water in a large saucepan and bring to a boil on high heat. Use 3 cups (705 ml) of water for a firmer consistency of grain, 3½ cups (825 ml) if you would prefer a porridge-like consistency, and 4 cups (946 ml) if you want a soup-like consistency. Add all of the remaining ingredients and stir. Then reduce the heat to low and simmer for 30–35 minutes covered. Stir occasionally and look for the desired consistency. Serve with sliced lemon, chopped cilantro, salt, and chutney to include all six tastes in one meal.

Note: Cooked kitchari congeals as it cools. If it congeals into a dense mass, reconstitute it to a pleasing texture simply by adding water and mashing it when you warm it up.

Breakfast Porridge and Konji

This whole-grain porridge is a staple breakfast for cleansing but is easy to prepare and enjoy in any season. You can modify the recipe for each type or season by choosing the appropriate grain, spice, and oil to deliver the necessary qualities. Konji is a thinner version of the porridge used in times of cleansing or weakness to make the food easier to digest. Konji can also be a healthy meal replacement or snack for busy times when the pace of your life makes it impossible to stop for a full meal.

YIELD • 3 CUPS (660 G) PORRIDGE; 4–6 CUPS (946–1425 ML) KONJI

1 cup (180 g) basmati rice or other grain

3 cups (705 ml) water (depending on the grain)

3 dates, soaked in water overnight and pitted

1 tablespoon (7 g) Sweet Milk spice mix (see page 86)

1 teaspoon ghee (2.3 g)

pinch of salt

squeeze of lemon

For konji:

additional 1–3 cups (235–705 ml) of water

One-pot cooking method: Combine the rice or grain and 2 cups (475 ml) of water in a large saucepan and cook on medium-high heat until the water boils. Reduce heat to low, stir, and simmer for 15 minutes. Add the remaining ingredients during the last few minutes of cooking, stir, and continue cooking until all the water is absorbed. Transfer to a blender, add the remaining 1 cup (235 ml) of water, and blend first on low, then on high for 1 minute until the porridge is creamy and smooth. Add more water if needed to achieve the desired consistency. The porridge should pour out of the blender when complete.

For konji: Use an additional 1–3 cups (235–705 ml) water to achieve a drinkable liquid. With more water it will resemble a nut milk or grain milk, but with less water it will be the consistency of a smoothie. In times of weak digestion or illness, use the thinner variety.

Caution: Leave the blender lid ajar or remove the round center insert when blending hot items. The heat will create expansion and pressure inside the blender and could cause the lid to pop off while blending.

Breeze: Use heavier grains like brown basmati rice for porridge when the digestive fire is strong. Drink konji when the digestive fire is weak.

Fire: Use basmati rice or quinoa for porridge and konji. Konji makes an ideal snack to satisfy hunger between meals.

Mountain: Use lighter grains like quinoa or millet and have konji for breakfast when lightening the diet.

Ghee (Clarified Butter)

Ayurveda considers ghee, or clarified butter, one of the most important food-medicines. When butter is heated, the thick and sticky milk solids separate from the clear, golden liquid that is ghee. You can strain the ghee out and use it in place of oil for cooking or as a garnish on grains, beans, or vegetables. It lubricates the digestive tract's mucous membranes, helps regulate digestion, lubricates the joints, and increases healthy cholesterol. Ghee is also used in Ayurveda to carry other herbal food-medicines deeper into the body, as ghee has the ability to penetrate into subtle and minute channels.

YIELD · APPROXIMATELY 2 CUPS (450 ML); YOU WILL LOSE A LITTLE GHEE WHEN STRAINING, SO IT IS USUALLY JUST SHORT OF 2 CUPS

1 pound (450 g) unsalted butter

Place the butter in a medium saucepan and warm on medium-low heat for 15–20 minutes. The milk solids will start to foam up on top of the clear liquid when the butter melts, and a bubbling sound will be audible as the water evaporates out of the butter. Around the 15-minute mark, the milk solids will start to sink and brown on the bottom of the pan. At this time, the bubbling sound will stop, signaling that the ghee is almost finished. A second foaming will happen after the ghee becomes quiet, but this foam has thin, clear bubbles opposed to the thick, white, chunky milk solids from the earlier stage. This is the proper time to remove the ghee from the heat. It is of utmost importance to watch the ghee carefully during this time, as it can burn within a minute if left on the heat after the process is complete.

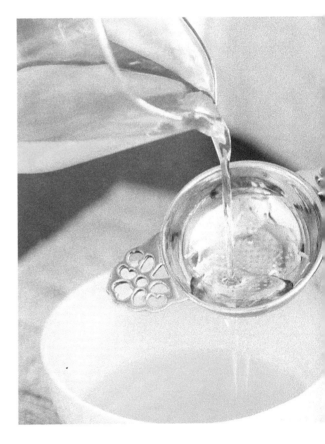

Remove the ghee from the heat and let it cool for 30 minutes. While it is still liquid, strain the ghee through a fine-mesh metal strainer or cheesecloth into a glass jar with a lid. Allow the ghee to cool and solidify completely before covering with the lid. You do not need to refrigerate the ghee as long as you keep moisture out of it. Use a clean, dry spoon each time you take ghee from the jar and then cover it immediately. Moisture in the ghee can allow bacteria to grow, so maintaining cleanliness is important.

Chutney

Chutney is a side dish or condiment served with savory dishes. Each of these recipes has all six tastes but is predominantly sweet in flavor to satiate the desire for sweet throughout the day. The fruit's sugar content acts as a preservative, so you can refrigerate a large batch of chutney for a week. The first chutney here is better for the Breeze, the second for the Mountain, and the third for Fire, but a small amount of any chutney is acceptable for all types.

YIELD • 1½ TO 2 CUPS (375–500 G) CHUTNEY

Raisin Coconut Chutney

1 cup (145 g) Thompson or flame raisins

½ cup (85 g) coconut

2 soaked and pitted dates

water, enough to cover fruits

1 teaspoon (2.3 g) ghee

1 teaspoon (2 g) fennel seed

pinch of salt

¼ teaspoon ground cardamom

¼ teaspoon ground ginger

squeeze of lemon

⅛ cup (7 g) chopped mint

Apple Cranberry Chutney

1 red or green apple, chopped

½ cup (60 g) dried cranberries

water, enough to cover fruits

1 teaspoon (2.3 g) ghee

1 teaspoon (2.1 g) whole cumin seed

¼ teaspoon ground cinnamon

pinch of salt

squeeze of lemon

⅛ cup (7 g) chopped parsley

1 teaspoon fresh grated ginger

Coconut Cilantro Chutney

½ cup (40g) shredded coconut

3 soaked and pitted dates

1 teaspoon (5 ml) coconut oil

1 teaspoon (2.1 g) whole cumin or fennel seed

½ cup (120 ml) coconut milk

½ cup (120 ml) water

pinch of salt

¼ teaspoon Sweet Milk spice (see page 86)

½ cup (8 g) chopped cilantro

For any of these recipes, place all dried and fresh fruits in a small saucepan and add just enough water to cover them. Simmer on medium-low heat uncovered for 15 minutes or until 90 percent of the water is absorbed. While the fruits are cooking, combine the ghee or oil and whole seeds in a small skillet and heat on low until the seeds start to brown and release their aroma (5–10 minutes). Turn off heat and combine the cooked fruits, roasted seeds, and all remaining ingredients in a blender or food processor. Blend on low for 30 seconds to 1 minute to make a chunky sauce. Serve warm in a colder season or cool for 20 minutes before serving in a warmer season. When using refrigerated chutney, take it out 30 minutes before a meal so that it can return to room temperature.

Caution: Leave the blender lid ajar or remove the round center insert when blending hot items. The heat will create expansion and pressure inside the blender and could cause the lid to pop off while blending.

Spice Mixes

Each spice mix is an appropriate blend for your type or your imbalance. You can use a mix with kitchari, individual grains or beans, soups, or vegetable mixes. If cooking for several individuals in your family with different body-mind types, use the Simple spice mix, which is tri-doshic. The first four blends are for use with savory dishes, and the Sweet Milk spice is for porridges, chutneys, or milk drinks.

YIELD • 24 SERVINGS, 1 OUNCE EACH

Warm the Breeze:

4 parts turmeric

3 parts coriander

2 parts cumin

2 parts ginger

1 part hing

Calm the Fire:

4 parts turmeric

3 parts coriander

3 parts cumin

2 parts fennel

Lift the Mountain:

4 parts turmeric

3 parts ginger

3 parts mustard seed

2 parts paprika

1 part cumin

1 part coriander

Simple:

3 parts turmeric

3 parts cumin

3 parts coriander

2 parts mustard seed

1 part hing

1 part ground ginger or

⅛ teaspoon freshly grated ginger per 1 tablespoon (7 g) of spice mix (added separately each time you prepare kitchari)

Sweet Milk:

4 parts cardamom

4 parts ginger (2 parts when used for the Fire)

1 part nutmeg

1 part cinnamon in warm weather; 2 parts in cold weather

Choose a spice mix and combine all ingredients together.

Each mix can be made in small or large batches and kept in a sealed container to preserve the potency of the spices. A small batch might use 1 teaspoon (2.4 g) per part, but a large batch might use ⅛ cup (14 g) per part.

Spiced Honey

Mountain individuals can use raw honey or raw, spiced honey as a sweetener for tea, warm milk, or porridge. Taken on an empty stomach, it is also good for clearing congestion from the lungs and sinuses in any body-mind type. Use spiced honey at the first sign of a cold to dry up excess secretion; for that purpose, take 1 teaspoon (6.5 g) once or twice daily.

YIELD • APPROXIMATELY 17 TEASPOONS (85g)

¼ cup (75 g) raw honey

1 tablespoon (5.5 g) ground ginger

1 teaspoon (2.3 g) ground cinnamon

1 teaspoon (2 g) ground black pepper or long pepper

½ teaspoon (1.2g) ground cardamom

Stir all ingredients thoroughly until all dry powders are coated with honey. Keep in a covered container and use a clean spoon with each use.

Note: Honey degenerates with high heat. Ancient Ayurveda taught that it becomes a toxic substance to the body when heated and advised against cooking with honey. When adding it to tea, allow the tea to cool for a few minutes first.

QUALITIES OF GINGER

The qualities of freshly grated ginger root are slightly different when it is dried or ground. The fresh root is sweeter and the dried root hotter. A small amount of fresh ginger is even safe for a Fire type when blended with other cooling spices. If the fresh root is available, use it in place of dried ginger in any recipe from this book. I alternate uses throughout the book because many people will not have access to the fresh variety.

Lemon-Ginger-Honey Nectar

This little zinger is always a favorite addition to any meal. The ingredients are all heating in nature, so together they stimulate the appetite and improve digestion. You can take nectar as a shot, 1 teaspoon to 1 ounce, (5–25 ml) before a meal or periodically throughout the day to help clear congestion in the lungs or sinuses.

Honey acts as a natural preservative, so I make a large batch and keep it refrigerated for a week or two. It is best to pour the shot and allow it to return to room temperature before serving. Eating or drinking anything colder than room temperature can weaken digestive fire and expend undue energy, because the body has to warm it up before assimilating it into the system.

You can prepare the nectar in different ratios for different individual needs. The standard recipe is three parts honey, two parts lemon juice, and one part ginger juice, but Mountain types can use equal amounts of honey, ginger juice, and lemon juice.

YIELD • 24 1-OUNCE (25 ML) SERVINGS

1-inch (2.5 cm) wide finger-length of ginger, grated or chopped

½ cup (120 ml) water

1 cup (240 ml) lemon juice

1½ cups (510 g) raw honey

Grate the ginger on a ceramic grater or chop in small pieces. If you have an industrial-grade blender, the size of the ginger chunks are not very important. If you have a standard blender, make the pieces of ginger as small as possible. Add the grated or chopped ginger to the blender with ½ cup of water. Blend on high and allow it to sit for 10 to 15 minutes. Blend again, then strain the ginger juice through a cheesecloth or fine-mesh metal strainer. Place the ginger juice, lemon juice, and raw honey in a jar and shake vigorously until the honey dissolves evenly. This may take several rounds of shaking.

Note: Use the remaining ginger pulp to make fresh ginger tea.

NAP FOR YOUR HEALTH

Improve the strength of your digestion by lying on your left side for fifteen to twenty minutes after a meal. This short "digestive nap" can help direct more energy to the body's natural process and increase the potency of the digestive juices in the stomach. Limit the nap to 20 minutes and you will wake up feeling refreshed!

TIPS FOR YOUR TYPE

Breeze: Use the standard recipe nectar and take 1 tablespoon to 1 ounce (15–25 ml) before meals.

Fire: Use the standard recipe nectar and take 1 teaspoon (5 ml) with breakfast and dinner during cleansing only.

Mountain: Use equal ratios in the nectar 1:1:1 and take 1 ounce (25 ml) before or after meals.

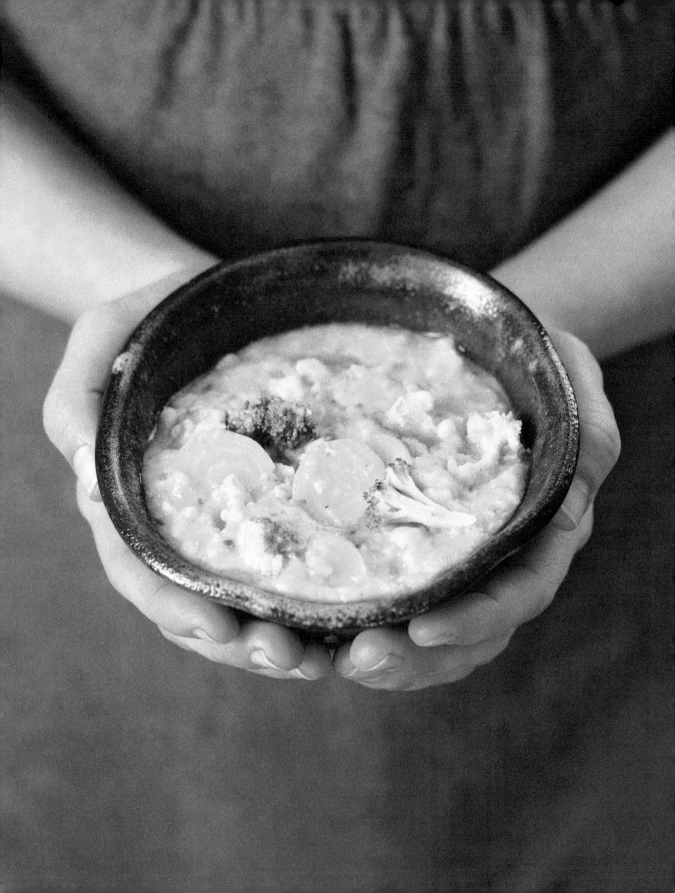

CHAPTER SIX

Grounding Cleanse & Diet

The purpose of this dietary cleanse is to gently lighten by consuming a vegetarian diet of whole grains, legumes, soaked nuts and seeds, fresh vegetables and fruits, good-quality oils and ghee, natural sweeteners, and warming spices. The diet is designed to be warming in nature, with well-cooked foods that are predominantly sweet, sour, and salty tastes. It is good for the Breeze constitution or those with a Breeze imbalance.

Daily practices and self-care include yoga poses, meditation, breath practices, and self-massage to calm the nervous system, relax the mind, ease stress, and create a sense of grounding. Use warming, heavy oils for self-massage to reduce the Breeze imbalance. Time away from the busyness and stresses of life is also advised, so that the nervous system can disengage, rest, and rebalance.

Daily Self-Care Practices

The self-care practices that best suit the Breeze individual are gentle. Remember the delicate flower in the meadow? Too much of anything—movement, touch, pressure, or cold—might damage her sensitive system. When taking on new practices, it is better for the Breeze individual to start gradually with one thing at a time, so that the practices can become a regular part of the daily routine during the 31-day protocol and beyond. Too many changes, too quickly will increase the Breeze imbalance instead of bringing balance.

Incorporate the following practices during the fourth week, along with the simple daily routine from chapter 5. These practices are gentle enough to be continued through the final three days of digestive cleansing for anyone, regardless of the cleanse chosen for week 4. They are also appropriate for everyday maintenance throughout the year for a Breeze type or an individual with a Breeze imbalance. Start with a practice that is interesting to you and commit to it for the entire week. If that feels easy, add another one. Continue in this manner and include as many of these practices as you can each day without increasing stress. Even a few minutes devoted to self-care breaks several times a day will make a difference.

Oil Self-Massage

The skin is the largest organ of the body, and every bit of it is intimately connected with nerve fibers, the extensions of the brain and nervous system. Like little fingers, these nerve fibers reach out to the skin to discover the world and respond to our interactions with it. These fibers carry signals for touch, pressure, pain, heat, and cold back to the brain, and each fiber is insulated with a fatty coating, the myelin sheath, which keeps the impulse contained and the delicate nerve protected. If the insulation—which acts like the plastic coating around an electrical wire—is dry, depleted, or thin, the nervous system can feel exposed and overly sensitive. Warm oil applied to the skin feels like putting a blanket of protection over the whole nervous system. It creates a sense of calm, stillness, stability, and grounding.

Ayurveda recommends a daily oil massage for everyone from the very first day of life to the last. The self-massage, called *Abhyanga*, focuses on long strokes over the long bones of the limbs to increase flow of blood and lymph and circular motions around the joints to release tension. The joints have a greater concentration of nerves, so the rhythmic circles applied with warm oil help to calm the nervous system. In fact, warm oil is one of the fastest ways to calm the whole nervous system.

Oils for Balance

Oil is a food-medicine for the body. It nourishes the skin and penetrates into the subtle channels to open any blockages in the tissues below. It can relieve aches and pains in the muscles with its penetrating action and improve overall circulation of fluids to aid in cleansing the body naturally. According to Ayurveda, the oil is absorbed through the skin and feeds the body in the same way food and water nourish through the digestive tract. It is important to realize that what you put on your skin is absorbed

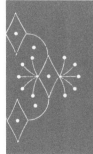

CONTRAINDICATIONS FOR OIL MASSAGE

The metabolic fire, agni, is also present on the cellular level in the body. It must be strong enough to digest the oil applied to the skin, otherwise it could result in the production of ama. For this reason, Ayurveda recommends avoiding oil application when the tongue has a thick coating, in acute illness, when fever is present, and during menstruation.

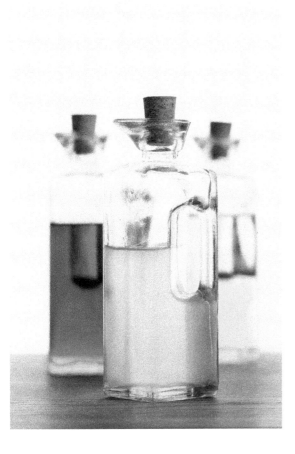

into the body. The common sense rule follows: If you would not put it in your mouth, do not put it on your skin.

Oil that is cold-pressed, organic, and processed without the use of chemicals is best for massage. The qualities of any oil are part of the nourishment and balance delivered through daily self-massage, so choose oil with this in mind. Herbalized oils are often used in Ayurveda to make a base oil more potent and more specific in its action.

- Breeze individuals need oils that are warming, calming, and grounding in nature, like sesame, olive, or almond oil. Herbalized vata oil has herbs to balance the Breeze and reduce vata. Ashwagandha Bala oil is a warming formula used for rejuvenation when high vata has depleted the tissues. Mahanarayan oil is a traditional formula that is appropriate for joint rejuvenation.

- Fire individuals need cooling and soothing oils such as coconut, sunflower, or safflower. Herbalized pitta oil has cooling herbs to balance the Fire and reduce pitta imbalances.

Fire types commonly use Brahmi oil in a coconut base for cooling and calming the mind.

- Mountain individuals require heating and stimulating oils like mustard or sesame. Herbalized kapha oil has herbs to balance the Mountain and reduce kapha accumulations. Mahanarayan oil also has properties that help remove congestion from the lungs and sinuses.

Quantity of oil for a massage varies, based on your constitution and current imbalance. Mountain individuals or those with naturally moist or oily skin can use one to two ounces (25–50 ml) per massage. Breeze individuals or those with dry skin can use up to eight ounces (200 ml). Fire individuals fall somewhere in the middle, so an average amount would be three to four ounces (75–100 ml) per massage.

Massage Setup and Procedure

Daily oil massage is the fountain of youth that will keep tissues soft, flexible, and healthy as we age. It is a simple practice, but is often set aside if the task of gathering supplies seems too difficult. Acquiring and organizing a few items and keeping them easily accessible will make self-massage easier.

Make sure you also have a warm space, such as your bathroom, where you can relax undressed and uninterrupted for ten to fifteen minutes while you are oiling. Any time of day or night is appropriate for massage, although morning is ideal for cleansing and evening is ideal for relaxing before bedtime. Make sure to allow adequate time so that you do not feel rushed through the process.

Note: Ayurveda recommends oiling before applying heat like a shower or bath, but I know individuals who have experienced serious problems with their plumbing due to oil. Consider oiling after bathing if you have sensitive plumbing. If you would prefer to leave the oil on your body throughout the day, first take a warm bath, shower, or steam to open the pores and then follow with your oil massage. Remember that some oil may get onto your clothing, so refer to the tips below for proper laundering.

TIPS FOR REMOVING OIL FROM CLOTH

In more than two decades of massage practice, I have used many products to aid in removing oil from towels, sheets, and clothing. I recommend Super Washing Soda by Arm & Hammer. When washing oily towels or sheets, use ¼ to ½ cup (55–115 g) washing soda in addition to your regular detergent and wash in hot water on a pre-soak cycle. To clean spots of oil from clothing, add a small amount of washing soda to your detergent and rub into the stain, then wash out in hot water. Use the dryer's low heat setting to dry our oil towels and sheets, to avoid combustion. You will eventually need to replace the towels when they feel oily or moist even after laundering.

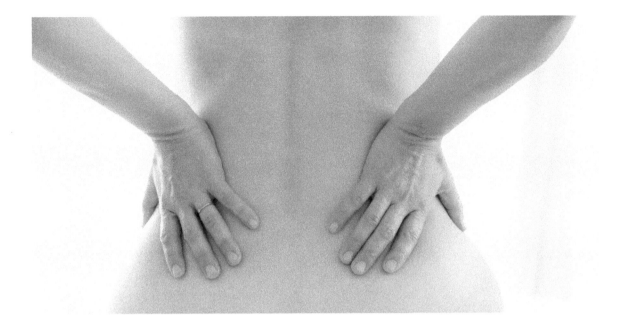

Oil Massage Instructions

1- to 8-ounces (25–200 ml) of oil appropriate for your type (see pages 93–94)

4- to 8-ounce (100–200 ml) plastic squeeze bottle or glass container with a well-sealed lid

small bowl

one or two old towels that can get oily

1. Place oil appropriate for your type in a four- to eight-ounce (100–200 ml) sealable glass container or plastic squeeze bottle. You also may want to have a small bowl available to hold and scoop oil after warming it.

2. Run hot water in your bathroom sink and place the oil bottle in the water for a few minutes. The oil should be comfortably warm when it is ready for application. Pour the proper amount of oil into the bowl to make application easy.

3. Place on old towel over a chair or on the floor to create a comfortable sitting area. Note: The towels will eventually build up oil, so dedicate a few old towels for daily massage and see left for how to launder properly.

4. Place a small amount of oil in your palm and apply it to your body. Start anywhere on your body that feels right and try to cover every bit of skin you can reach. It is more important to focus on the speed and intention of your touch than the mechanics or details of the massage. Move slowly for calming (Breeze and Fire types) or vigorously for stimulating (Mountain

types), and focus on giving love to each part of your body. The Ayurvedic word for "oil," sneha, is also the word for "love."

5. Apply the oil with long up-and-down strokes on your limbs and circular motions around the joints. Use circular clockwise motions at the navel, circular motions on the chest and around breasts, and long up-and-down strokes along the spine (as much as you can reach with your hands behind your back). Massage each finger and toe thoroughly.

6. Pour 1- to 4-ounces (25–100 ml) of oil on the top of your head and spread it around

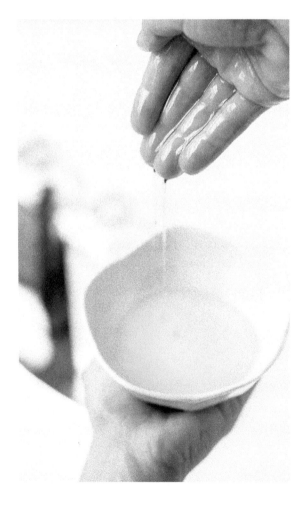

your scalp. Use more oil if you are in need of calming the nervous system or slowing down the mind and less oil if you are feeling heavy, dull, or congested. Lean forward and massage your whole scalp with shampooing movements of your fingers. While bending forward, rest your elbows on your thighs or knees so that your shoulders will not feel tired or strained from the work of massaging. Massage your face and neck using the whole palm to relax tight muscles with special focus on the front and sides of your neck.

7. Relax in the warm room for a few minutes with the oil on your skin.

8. Pat off excess oil with an old towel and make sure your feet are not slippery. (If you are leaving the oil on for the rest of the day, skip step 9.)

9. Take a warm bath, steam, or shower, being extremely careful not to slip. The warm water opens your pores and allows the oil to penetrate deeper into your tissues. It is not necessary to soap your skin, but you can use a mild soap on your hairy parts. If you want to wash your hair, it is best to apply the shampoo directly to your oiled hair before wetting it. This will allow the oil and shampoo to bond, so that the oil will rinse out easily.

10. Take a few minutes to be still, breathe deeply, and notice the effects of the oil massage on your body and mind. The manner in which you start or end your day will set the tone physically and emotionally for everything that follows. A relaxing massage experience in the morning can help you maintain calm throughout the day; before bedtime, it can bring sound, restful sleep.

Breathing Practices

The deep belly breath and the three-part breath are the foundational steps to all other breathing practices. These are the natural breaths we use as babies and the pattern of breathing we return to in sleep. It brings calming and grounding by sending a signal to the nervous system that it is safe to relax. But in waking hours, the effects of stress, emotional blockages, and constriction of muscles around the rib cage often make our breathing shallow.

The three-part breath, or long breath, is often easier to accomplish lying down at first, but with practice can be done in any position, at any time. Ideally, it is the breath we use every moment of every day. I recommend starting with part 1 and practicing until that is comfortable, then adding the other two parts. Use this breath for a few minutes in bed before sleeping and after waking, and then take breaks throughout the day to remind your body to stay calm.

Sit or lie down in a comfortable position. Notice your breath. Allow it to become slow and deep.

Part 1: Inhale and invite the breath down into your belly and let the lower abdomen (below the navel) expand in all directions, then exhale fully. Expand the space in and around the hips, genitals, and low back, filling the entire bowl of your pelvis with breath. After several long, slow, deep belly breaths, allow the breath to expand upward, toward the lower rib cage.

Part 2: Expand the belly first and then the lower rib cage with each inhalation. You can place one hand on the belly and one on the lower ribs to draw your attention there. As you exhale, try to allow the rib area to let go first, then the belly. Continue for several breaths.

Part 3: Now let the breath move up the body like a wave: Inhale into the belly first, the lower ribs second, and finally into the upper ribs, just below the collarbone, so that the chest lifts. Now allow the wave of breath to flow out from the upper ribs, then from the lower ribs, followed by the belly. Finally, squeeze the navel to the spine to press out all the air. Continue with this breath for several minutes.

Meditation

Meditation is a practice to reconnect with the natural and healthy state of the mind—stable, calm, clear, and pure—to witness the true self within. The first step in learning to meditate is concentration exercises to make the mind one-pointed. Tratakam, or candle-gazing, is a concentration practice that can become a meditation. This is an ideal starting place for those new to meditation and also for people with an active imagination or mind who may get lost in their own thoughts with a closed-eye meditation. Practice for a few minutes at a time.

Sit in a comfortable position. Watch the flame of a burning candle. Let your awareness become pointed on the flame. If any thoughts arise in the mind, notice them, but return your attention to the flame. Keep a relaxed body and breath without giving too much attention to either.

Notice if it is easy to still the mind and remain focused or if the mind's activity keeps taking you away from the flame. Continue to watch both the flame and whatever arises in you from the perspective of a witness, as if you were watching a movie. Remind yourself compassionately to bring your awareness back to the flame again and again. Use this practice regularly to create a calm, still, and single-pointed focus in the mind.

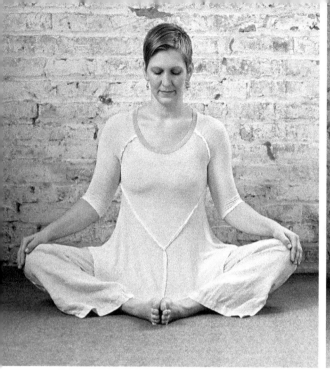

Bound angle

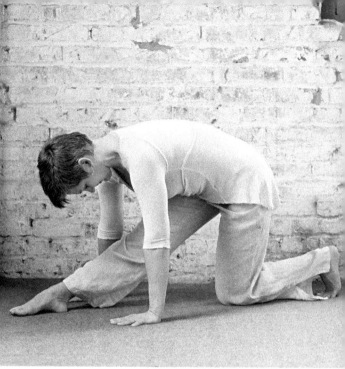

Forward bend

Yoga Poses

Yoga postures for balancing the Breeze are calm, steady, slow, grounding, strengthening, warming, and consistent. They stretch and open the spine, low back, hips, back of the legs, and joints. These include seated positions, forward bending postures, gentle movements of the spine and joints, hip openers, and reclining postures. Gentle backbends while lying down can strengthen the low back and core muscles, as can standing postures that focus on grounding.

Precautions: Forward-bending postures can create excess pressure on herniated or bulging discs in the spine or on the vertebrae when osteoporosis is present. To prevent this, bend forward from the hips, with a straight spine.

Try these three postures individually or together:

Joint Circles

Rotate each joint in circles slowly (ten times in each direction) to create more range of motion and produce more synovial fluid for ease of movement. You can do this in a reclining, seated, or standing position. Include the ankles, knees, hips, wrists, elbows, shoulder, and neck, but note that the knees and elbows will only bend and straighten. Be careful with the neck: Forward bending is safe, but backward movement may pinch nerves of the spine or compress vertebrae. Circle the neck, but bring the head straight across from one shoulder to the other (not backward).

Bound Angle, or the Butterfly Posture

Sit on the floor with your legs crossed. If your low back rounds outward or feels tight, sit on a cushion, folded blanket, or a block, so that you can sit up straight. Place the soles of the feet together and let the knees drop out to the sides. If there is strain in the knees, place a pillow under each one for support.

Take a few deep belly breaths and allow the hips and thighs to relax. If this is comfortable, then "flap your butterfly wings" by raising and lowering the knees simultaneously. Return to stillness, then lean forward with a straight back until you feel a stretch in the low back and hips. Breathe deeply and lengthen the spine as you inhale, then sink down deeper into the stretch as you exhale. Finally, allow your back to round as you curl over the legs, finding the stretch that is just right for you, using your hands on the ground for support. Relax here and continue deep belly breaths, then slowly come out of the stretch.

Lunge to Forward Bend

Start in a kneeling position with your torso upright. If your knees are tender, place a blanket under them for padding. Step your right foot forward and place the sole of your foot on the floor in front of you, taking a lunge position (see page 98). Rock forward and backward in this position, feeling the hips opening.

Bend forward and round over the right leg, letting your hands come to the floor for support. (If your hands do not touch the floor, use two yoga blocks—one on each side of the right leg—for hand supports.) Take a few deep breaths and feel the muscles along the spine stretch. Begin to straighten the right (front) leg gently and then release the stretch by bending the knee. Allow your whole body to rock with these alternating movements. Finally, straighten the leg and relax into the stretch along the entire back of the body, including the calf, hamstring, low back, and spine. Breathe deeply and

hold for one minute, then slowly release. Repeat this sequence with the other leg.

Tips for Successful Dietary Cleansing

These recommendations are geared toward an individual with a Breeze constitution or a Breeze imbalance, to improve health and balance on a daily basis. They are also particularly important during the week of dietary cleansing and the final three days of digestive cleansing. After you have completed the first three weeks of the 31-day protocol and move into the fourth week, follow these suggestions as much as possible.

Meals: Drink a warming tea thirty minutes before each meal and take lemon-ginger-honey nectar (see page 67) immediately before each meal to improve appetite and digestive fire. Take a nap afterward to support the process of digestion (see page 67).

Snacks: If you are hungry between meals, choose cooked fruit with warming spices, warm milk drinks, or warm konji and make sure to allow proper time (thirty minutes for fruit alone; two hours for konji) to digest the snack before your next meal.

Water: Drink only warm water this week. Start your day with a large glass of warm water with lemon, and take self-care breaks to drink water periodically throughout the day—one hour before or two hours after a meal. Reduce water intake in the evening hours, so that it does not interfere with sound sleep.

Rest: Try to be in bed by 9:30 p.m., so that you can be asleep by 10. Make a goal of eight full hours of sleep each night, and try to rise between 6 and 7 a.m.. If your sleep is disturbed during the night, use calming practices from the self-care section to create enough grounding to return to sleep (see pages 69 to 77).

Self-care: Prioritize an evening self-care routine so that heaviness can accumulate in the body and prepare it for sleep. Oil the body at night and then take a warm bath if you have any challenges staying asleep. Oil both morning and night if you have the time and your tongue is free of excess coating. Incorporate as many practices as you can in the morning and at night without feeling rushed. If necessary, stay warm with extra layers of clothing.

Stress-reduction: If you can, take time away from work during this week; the more that you can relax the nervous system, the better your results from the cleanse will be. If not, take self-care breaks periodically during the day to practice deep breaths, yoga poses, or meditation; even five minutes will help. Prioritize the deep breathing exercises as the most important practice every day.

"eat more" list
— for the breeze's daily diet and the grounding cleanse —

Choose foods that are **warm, moist, heavy, and oily** in quality and tastes that are **sweet, sour, and salty**.

Eat more of the following:

fruits that are sweet, sour, heavy, or juicy in nature, such as avocadoes, bananas, berries, cherries, figs, grapefruit, grapes, lemons, mangoes, sweet melons,

Daily Schedule

6-7 a.m.	Wake, ideally after eight hours of sleep.
	Do deep belly breaths.
	Drink warm water.
	Eliminate waste from bowels and bladder.
	Do yoga poses.
	Clean the senses; observe the tongue.
	Oil and shower (now or at night; both if time allows).
7:30 a.m.	Drink tea.
8 a.m.	Breakfast.
11 a.m.	Self-care break with deep breaths or yoga poses, followed by water intake.
Noon	Drink tea.
12:30 p.m.	Lunch (your biggest and heaviest meal), followed by a digestive nap (see page 67).
4 p.m.	Self-care break with deep breaths or yoga poses, followed by water intake.
5:30 p.m.	Drink tea.
6 p.m.	Dinner.
8:30 p.m.	Do yoga poses or oil and take a warm bath; do candle-gazing meditation, and put drops of oil in ears.
9:30 p.m.	Consume warm milk drink and prepare for bedtime; go to sleep by 10 p.m.

oranges, lemons, limes, papayas, peaches, pineapples, and plums. Most fruits are good for the Breeze individual. Cooked fruits are better in a cold season or when the digestive fire is weak.

vegetables that are sweet or heavy in nature, such as asparagus, beets, carrots, cucumbers, garlic, green beans, okra, cooked onions, parsnips, peas, sweet potatoes, yellow squash, zucchini, and yams. *Eat in moderation*: lettuce, leafy greens, sprouts, and spinach. *Eat well cooked*, with oil and proper spices: broccoli, Brussels sprouts, cabbage, cauliflower, celery, kale, potatoes, tomatoes, and winter squashes.

grains that are heavy or warming, such as basmati rice, brown rice, wild rice, oats, quinoa, and wheat

legumes that are easy to digest, such as mung beans, soy, and yellow or red lentils

nuts and seeds if they are soaked, made into nut milks, or cooked, especially almonds and sesame seeds

ghee or raw cow's milk as food-medicines for lubrication and nourishment, if you eat dairy

oils of sesame, olive, and almond

sweeteners that are natural and unprocessed, such as raw sugar, molasses, rice syrup, and, in moderation, honey and maple syrup

condiments that are warming, sweet, sour, or salty, such as basil, lemon, lime, salt, seaweed, and vinegar, and, occasionally, cilantro or mint

spices that are sweet, warming, and calming in nature such as cardamom, curry leaves, ginger, fenugreek, and hing. Use coriander, cumin, fennel, saffron, or turmeric in combination with other warming spices and use cinnamon and nutmeg in moderation.

For non-cleansing times, use mushroom broths or bone broths, (if you consume animal products) to build strength—or beef, chicken, or turkey.

Limit or avoid the following types of foods:

- cold, dry, or light in nature
- astringent, bitter, and pungent in taste
- rough and dry such as crackers, chips, or popcorn
- raw, cold, rough, and difficult-to-digest foods, including raw fruits, vegetables, and nuts (except in a warm season or when you are making them into juice or milk)

GROUNDING RECIPES

The recipes that follow include foods that are warm, well cooked, moist, and oily, to counter the cold, dry, and light qualities of Breeze and create a lighter workload for a delicate digestive fire. The ingredients are mostly calming in nature, with a few stimulating spices and vegetables like onions and garlic used to create more warmth. The spice blends kindle the digestive fire, the heavier root vegetables create a warm and grounded feeling, and whole grains and legumes provide a complete protein that is easy to digest. These recipes are best for the autumn as part of a seasonal diet, throughout the year for those with a Breeze constitution or imbalance, or as part of the grounding dietary cleanse.

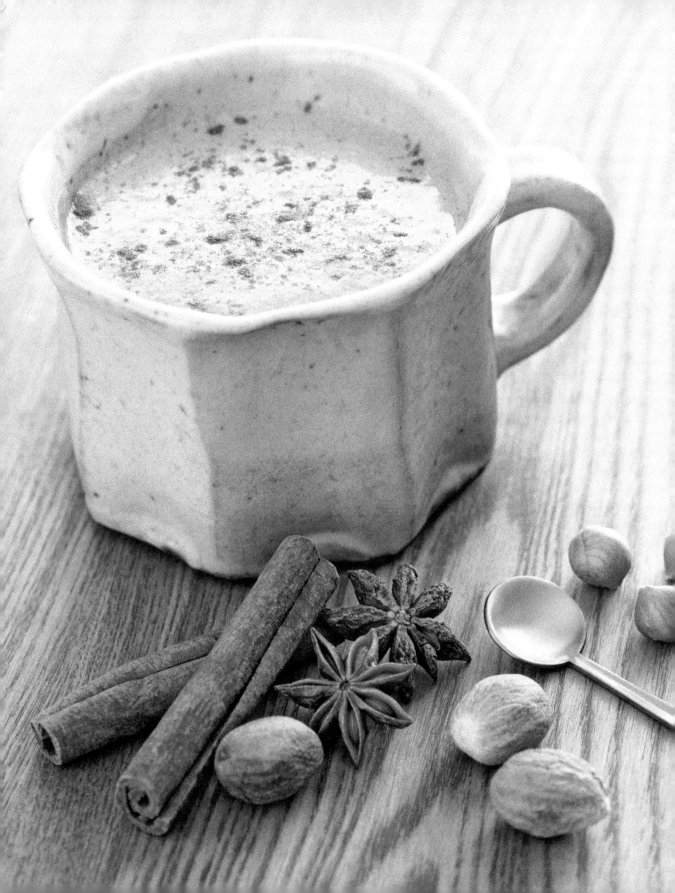

Indian Chocolate Spice

Enjoy all the creamy deliciousness of the richest hot chocolate—without the guilt. Since there is no chocolate in this recipe, the magic ingredient here is the powdered root ananta mula, nicknamed "Indian Chocolate" for its rich, earthy, sarsaparilla-spiced flavor. The root's heavy, grounding qualities nourish deeply while satiating the desire for sweet. Combined with warming spices, this drink is perfect as an evening ritual before bedtime or a hand-and-heart-warming answer to the cold of fall.

YIELD • 2 SERVINGS, ½ CUP (120 ML) EACH

1 cup (235 ml) raw cow's milk, fresh almond milk, or hazelnut milk

1 tablespoon (7 g) ananta-mula powder

¼ teaspoon (1.8 g) ginger powder

¼ teaspoon (2 g) cardamom powder

¼ teaspoon (2.3 g) cinnamon powder

⅛ teaspoon (2.2 g) nutmeg powder

1 star anise, whole

1 teaspoon (5 g) ghee

maple syrup to taste

Combine the milk, ananta-mula powder, and spices in a small saucepan and warm on medium heat for 5 to 7 minutes until it starts to gently boil and foam. Remove from the heat, scoop out the star anise, add the ghee, and mix in a blender first on low, then on medium-high. Pour ½-cup to 1-cup (120–235 ml) servings into mugs. Add maple syrup if more sweet taste is desired.

Caution: Make sure the blender lid is secure, because the heat will cause expansion and pressure inside the blender and could pop the lid off.

TIPS FOR YOUR TYPE

Fire: Cut spice amounts in half.

Mountain: Use almond or hazelnut milk, add a pinch of black pepper, and omit sweetener and ghee. Drink in moderation.

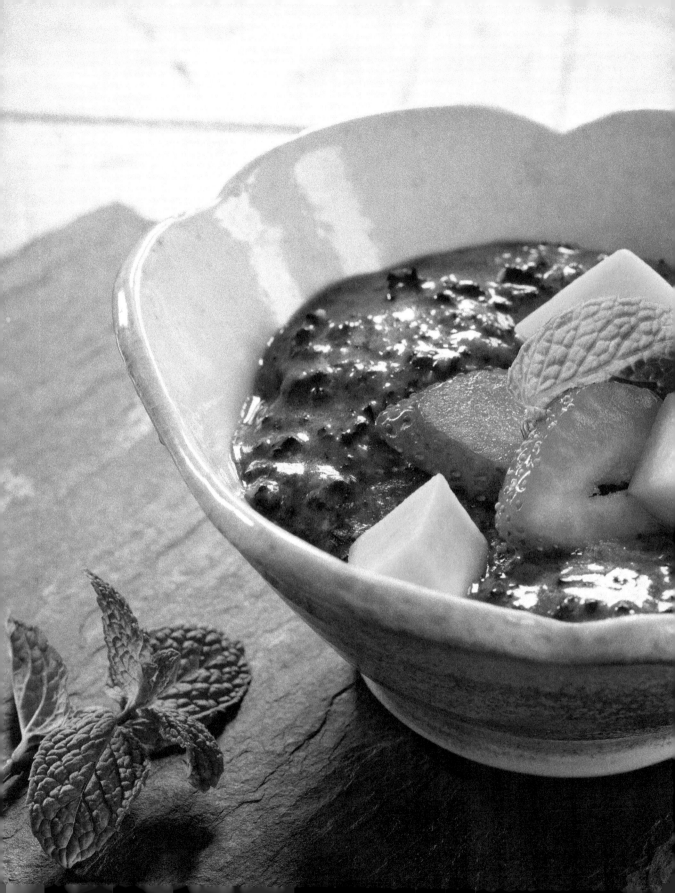

Black Rice and Cashew Porridge

Chewy, creamy, and delicious! My husband tasted a porridge made with forbidden black rice at one of our favorite breakfast places, Haven, in Lenox, Massachusetts. He raved about it for so long that I finally had to try making it. The black rice was perfect—a firm texture that turns chewy, yet creamy when cooked and blended. It is definitely my favorite version of breakfast porridge.

YIELD • THREE TO FOUR ¾- OR 1-CUP (165–220 G) SERVINGS; 3½ CUPS (770 G) TOTAL

3 cups (706 ml) water

pinch of salt

1 cup (190 g) black rice, uncooked

¼ cup (50 g) cashews, soaked

¼ teaspoon (0.6 g) ground cardamom

1 cup (235 ml) oat or almond milk

1 teaspoon (5 g) ghee

4 dates, soaked overnight in water and pitted

For garnish:

fresh sliced strawberries or mango with mint or cooked apples and pears (see page 170)

Place 2½ cups (580 ml) water and salt in a medium saucepan and bring to a boil on high heat. Add the rice, reduce heat to low, and simmer, covered, for 20 minutes or until all of the water is absorbed. Transfer the rice into a blender and add all other ingredients, plus an additional ½ cup (120 ml) hot water. Blend on low, then high, until porridge is creamy and well blended. To serve, pour into bowls and garnish with your choice of fresh sliced fruit or cooked fruit.

Caution: Leave the blender lid ajar or remove the round center insert when blending hot items. The heat will create expansion and pressure inside the blender and could cause the lid to pop off while blending. You can also blend smaller portions to ensure your safety.

Note: If your digestion is weak, eliminate the fresh-fruit garnish and eat raw fruit only when it is ripe and in season.

TIPS FOR YOUR TYPE

Fire: Choose cooked apples and pears as a garnish.

Mountain: Use additional water instead of milk; do not use ghee or dates (use spiced honey for additional sweetness); choose cooked apples and pears as a garnish; and enjoy only occasionally.

Gingery Oatmeal Squares with Banana-Berry Delight Sauce

I originally tried a breakfast oatmeal bar at Café Azafran in Delaware. I decided to make a lighter version without eggs, sugar, or heavy dairy products. I incorporated tips I have used in the past when cooking for vegan friends, using bananas and dates as the glue that holds it all together. The flaxseeds also add a slippery quality that helps lubricate the digestive tract and ease the movement of the bowels. It's a perfect warm, nourishing breakfast for the Breeze or during the fall.

YIELD • EIGHT 2-INCH (5 CM) SQUARES

Dry ingredients

2 cups (160 g) rolled oats, uncooked

⅓ cup (56 g) flaxseeds

⅓ cup (37 g) almond meal

⅓ cup (40 g) oat flour

½ teaspoon (1.2 g) ground cinnamon

1 teaspoon (1.8 g) ground ginger

pinch of salt

Wet ingredients

2 tablespoons (28 g) ghee, melted

1 tablespoon (21 g) maple syrup

1 teaspoon (5 ml) vanilla extract

2 ripe bananas

4 soaked and pitted dates

½ cup (120 ml) oat milk

For sauce:

1 ripe banana, sliced

2 cups (145 g) sweet berries, any variety

¼ cup (120 ml) water

Combine all dry ingredients in a large bowl or food processor and mix. Add wet ingredients and mix again. If hand-mixing, you may want to puree the bananas, dates, and oat milk in a blender first. Use coconut oil or ghee to grease an 8-inch by 8-inch (20-cm by 20-cm) pan, then spread the oat mixture into the pan and bake on 350°F (Gas Mark 4) for 25–30 minutes. The top of the bars should appear browned and a little crusty when done. Let cool for 10 minutes and cut into squares.

For sauce: Place all ingredients in a small saucepan and cook on medium heat for 15 minutes, stirring occasionally. The sauce will continue to thicken as more water evaporates, so cook less if you want a juicy sauce or more for a thicker sauce.

To serve: Place one or two oat squares in a bowl and pour oat milk on it and warm banana-berry sauce over the top.

Note: The oat squares also make a great snack with Apricot Cherry Sauce (see page 103).

TIPS FOR YOUR TYPE

Fire: Use half the amount of ginger and substitute coconut oil or coconut butter for ghee.

Mountain: Use the Apricot Cherry Sauce (see page 103) instead of the Banana Berry Delight sauce and eat this only occasionally, as the ingredients are heavy, sweet, moist, sticky, and building to the tissues.

TIPS FOR YOUR TYPE

Fire: Eat in moderation, as the beets can be heating.

Mountain: Add 2 extra cups (480 ml) of water to make the soup thinner; add black pepper; and omit ghee.

Golden Glow Soup

Golden beets are a special treat: a burst of yellow sunshine with a milder flavor than their deep-red cousins. The glow of the beets is enhanced by turmeric, a golden root resembling ginger but with a dark-orange internal flesh, that is commonly dried, ground, and used as a spice in Indian cuisine. For centuries Indian women have used turmeric as their beauty secret for youthful, glowing skin.

YIELD · SIX 1-CUP (250 G) SERVINGS

½ leek, chopped

1 tablespoon (14 g) ghee

2 medium golden beets, peeled and chopped

6 medium potatoes, chopped

1-inch (2.5 cm) piece turmeric root, grated, or 1 tablespoon (6.8 g) ground turmeric

1 teaspoon (2.5 g) ground cumin

1 teaspoon (6 g) salt

1 quart (946 ml) water

For garnish:

1 tablespoon (1 g) chopped cilantro

Add the leek and ghee to a large soup pot and sauté on medium-low for 5 minutes. Add the remaining ingredients and cook on medium-high for 20 minutes or until the vegetables are soft. Pour into blender and puree. Transfer into bowls and garnish with chopped cilantro.

Caution: Leave the blender lid ajar or remove the round center insert when blending hot items. The heat will create expansion and pressure inside the blender and could cause the lid to pop off while blending. You can also blend smaller portions to ensure your safety.

ADD IT!

For a beautiful splash of color and flavor when you are not cleansing, add a garnish of red beet juice or red beet puree mixed with goat cheese.

1 small red beet, juiced • ¼ cup (35 g) goat cheese

For garnish: Wash, peel, and juice one red beet, then mix with goat cheese. Pour over individual servings of soup and sprinkle cilantro on top.

Alternately, if you do not have a juicer, chop one-half of a red beet and place in a small saucepan with just enough water to cover it. Cook for 15–20 minutes or until the beets are soft, then pour into a blender with the goat cheese and puree.

What Do I Have in the Kitchen?
Water-Sautéed Veggies

Adding water to a sauté is a technique to combine the moist and soft qualities of steaming with the oily qualities of sautéing. This is ideal for the Breeze who needs moist, soft, oily foods that are well cooked. This technique can also help reduce the amount of oil used to cook foods. A small amount of water adds a slippery quality that can take the place of additional oil, so this can help the Fire and Mountain types when they are limiting oil to lighten or cleanse the body. Use any combination of vegetables you find in the kitchen.

YIELD • FOUR 1-CUP (135 G) SERVINGS

10 Brussels sprouts, halved

4 small orange carrots, peeled and chopped into 1-inch (3 cm) coins

4 small purple carrots, peeled and chopped into 1-inch (2.5 cm) coins

1 teaspoon (5 g) ghee or oil

2 tablespoons (28 ml) water

pinch of salt

¼ teaspoon ground ginger or ¼-inch piece fresh ginger, grated

¼ teaspoon ground coriander

squeeze of lemon or splash of vinegar

Combine chopped vegetables, ghee or oil, and water in a medium sauté pan and cook on medium heat until the water starts to steam. Cover with a lid, reduce heat to low, and cook for 10–15 minutes until all of the water is absorbed and the vegetables are tender to your liking. Add the salt, spices, and lemon or vinegar in the last few minutes of cooking and stir the vegetables to coat evenly. Remove from heat and serve.

Tips: If you are chopping vegetables for the sauté that are different densities, like Brussels sprouts and green beans, start with the hardest ones first. Start heating the oil and water when you begin chopping and add the vegetables as you chop them. This way the Brussels sprouts get more time cooking and the green beans get less.

TIPS FOR YOUR TYPE

Fire: Use cooling ingredients such as kale and coconut oil.

Mountain: Use lighter vegetables that are bitter and pungent in taste, such as chard and radishes; add more heating spices like black pepper and paprika; use less ghee or use mustard oil as a substitute; and do not cover with a lid, so that the vegetables retain less moisture.

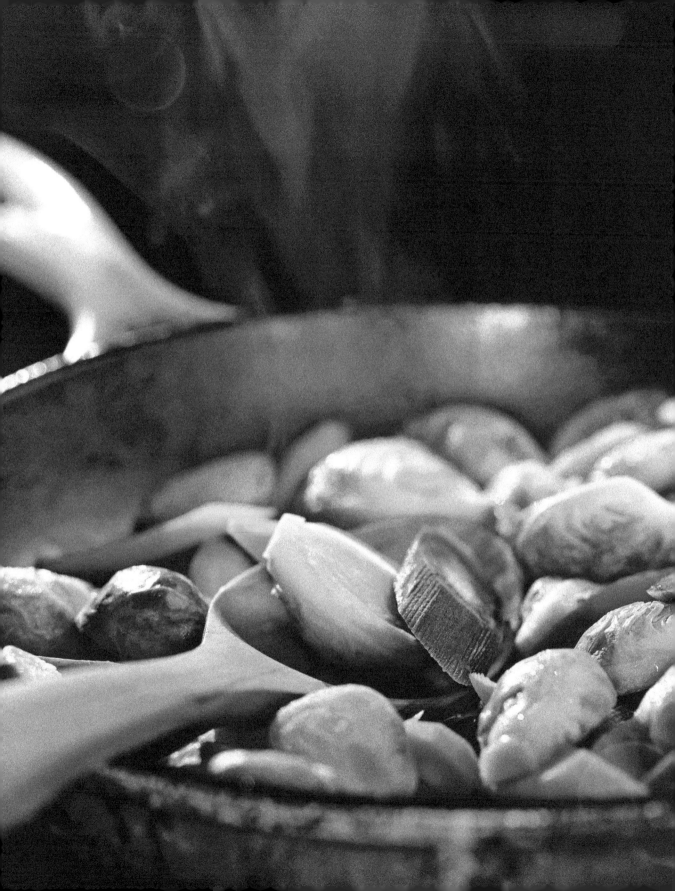

Belly-Warming Curried Roots with Tamarind Sauce

This is a great fall warmer, when soft comfort foods are appealing. I like to chop the vegetables into large pieces when I make this as a main dish with lemon rice or another grain, but I chop them into tiny pieces when I plan on mixing them with kitchari. Fenugreek, hing, and turmeric make for a powerful digestive aid that can remove excess vata, dispel gas, and remove toxins from the gastrointestinal tract. You can also use this spice mix when cooking beans, to reduce gas and bloating that are common with poor digestion. My belly always feels warm and happy after a meal with curried roots!

YIELD · FOUR 1½-CUP (270 G) SERVINGS

¼ cup (60 ml) water

2 tablespoons (28 ml) olive oil

6 fresh curry leaves, diced

¼ teaspoon ground fenugreek

¼ teaspoon ground turmeric

¼ teaspoon asafoetida (hing)

1 cup (110 g) chopped parsnips

1 cup (150 g) chopped yams

6 pearl onions or shallots, peeled and chopped

1 cup (225 g) chopped beets, any varieties

½ cup (50 g) chopped fennel root

1 cup (130 g) chopped tricolor carrots

For garnish:
fresh basil leaves

For sauce:

4 tablespoons wet tamarind paste

1 cup (235 ml) hot water

1 teaspoon (2.6 g) ground fennel

1 teaspoon (1.8 g) ground ginger

1 teaspoon (2.5 g) ground cumin

⅛ teaspoon ground paprika

⅛ teaspoon chili powder

¼ teaspoon (1.5 g) salt

2 tablespoons (42 g) maple syrup

squeeze of lemon

Mix water, oil, curry leaves, and spices in the bottom of a glass baking dish or covered clay baking pot. Add all chopped vegetables and coat thoroughly in the oil and spice mixture. Bake at 400°F (204°C) for 30–40 minutes, stirring occasionally to recoat the vegetables. In an uncovered baking dish, the vegetables will have a dry and roasted appearance when done and will be fork-tender—better for the Mountain types. When baked in a covered dish, the vegetables will be steamed with a softer and slightly mushy texture, which is better for the Breeze. Baking time will vary; 30 minutes is adequate for finely chopped vegetables, while larger chunks will require 40 minutes or longer. Garnish with fresh basil leaves.

For sauce: Pour hot water over wet tamarind paste and soak for a few minutes. Stir and press the paste with a spoon or hand to separate the fruit from the seeds and hair-like particles. Combine all other ingredients in a small bowl and strain the tamarind through a fine mesh strainer into the bowl. Press the pulp into and through the strainer and mix the ingredients thoroughly. Pour over individual servings to taste.

TIPS FOR YOUR TYPE

Fire: Omit onions, black pepper, or ginger if they cause discomfort.

Mountain: In the marinade, use tahini instead of cashew butter, lemon instead of orange, sesame oil instead of olive oil, and an extra ¼ teaspoon each of paprika, ginger, and black pepper. Bake the tofu for an extra 5 minutes to reduce the moisture and heaviness.

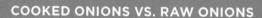

COOKED ONIONS VS. RAW ONIONS

Onions are hot, sharp, and tend to aggravate or increase the Fire imbalance. However, cooking onions brings out their natural sweetness, rendering them easier for the Fire type to tolerate. Cooked onions are okay for the Fire type in moderation, but I have encountered more than one Fire individual who could not tolerate even these. So listen to your own body, and if you feel any burning or digestive discomfort after ingesting onions, leave them out next time.

Beans and Greens with Cashew Miso Tofu

Tofu is an easy way to add a little excitement to a simple meal of staples. I think many people avoid tofu because they do not know how to prepare it. It will take on the flavor of any sauce, so the only trick to delicious tofu is to create an interesting marinade. Even before I studied Ayurveda, I noticed that I was relying on three tastes when creating a marinade: sweet, sour, and salty. Now I add a hint of pungent to aid digestion.

YIELD • FOUR 1½-CUP (270 G) SERVINGS

1 cup (192 g) lentils or adzuki beans, soaked in water

3 cups (706 ml) water

½ cup (72 g) corn

10 pearl onions

½ cup (70 g) finely chopped carrots

1 teaspoon (2.7 g) grated ginger

1 teaspoon (5 g) ghee

½ teaspoon (3.5 g) salt

For water-sauté:

1 cup (100 g) chopped bok choy

1 cup (100 g) chopped green beans

½ cup (150 g) green peas

2 teaspoons (10 ml) water

¼ teaspoon (1.3 ml) olive oil

For tofu:

15 ounces (425 g) tofu, drained and pressed

1 tablespoon (15 g) cashew butter or tahini

1 teaspoon (5.3 g) miso

1 orange, squeezed

1 tablespoon (15 ml) liquid aminos

2 tablespoons (30 ml) olive oil

pinch of paprika and black pepper

Soak the lentils or adzuki beans in water overnight, drain, and place in a medium stockpot with three cups water. Cook on high heat until the water boils, then reduce heat to low, cover, and simmer for 30 minutes. Add all remaining ingredients, stir, and cook for another 20–25 minutes or until the beans and vegetables are soft and tender. While the beans are cooking, water-sauté the vegetables in a medium skillet with a lid (see page 88).

For the tofu: Drain the water from the tofu, then slice into three ½-inch (1.3 cm) rectangular slabs. Place one clean towel under the tofu on a cutting board or hard surface and another towel over the tofu. Use a large cookbook to press down firmly and evenly on the tofu for 1 minute, then allow it to stay pressed with the weight of the cookbook for another 10 minutes. To create the marinade, mix the remaining ingredients in a small bowl or on a plate with a rim. Slice the tofu into 1-inch (2.5 cm) strips, soak in the marinade for 5 minutes, then bake in the oven for 20 minutes at 375°F (190°C).

To serve: Ladle ½- to 1-cup (about 90–180 g) servings of beans into a bowl, cover with ½-cup (about 70 g) serving of greens, and top with 4 or 5 strips of baked tofu.

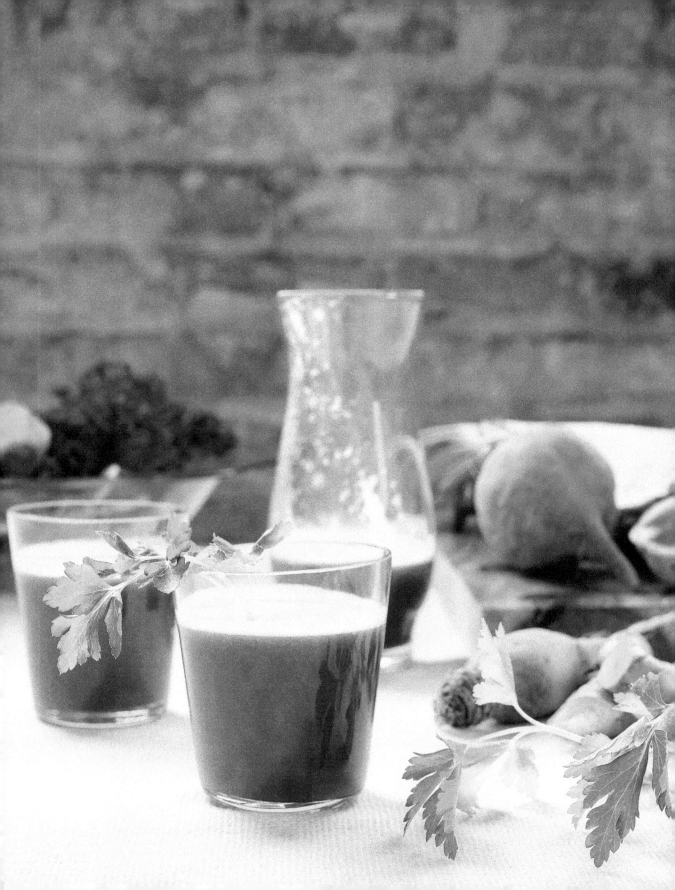

CHAPTER SEVEN

Lightening Cleanse & Diet

The purpose of this dietary cleanse is to use stimulating, heating, and reducing practices and foods to lighten the body. The foods consumed are light, dry, and heating in nature with predominantly pungent, bitter, and astringent tastes. The vegetarian diet consists of light and astringent whole grains, legumes, light seeds, and abundant vegetables prepared with heating spices. Oils, fats, salt, fruits, and honey are used sparingly. This cleanse is appropriate for an individual with a Mountain constitution or a Mountain imbalance.

The practices for self-care and daily maintenance include stimulating yoga poses, breathing practices, and vigorous exercise to induce sweating. Heat from the sun, dry sauna, steam, or shower is advisable to create movement and dry up excess secretions. Finally, dry massage with raw silk gloves improves circulation and lymphatic movement to help in cleansing. These practices are all lightening and reducing.

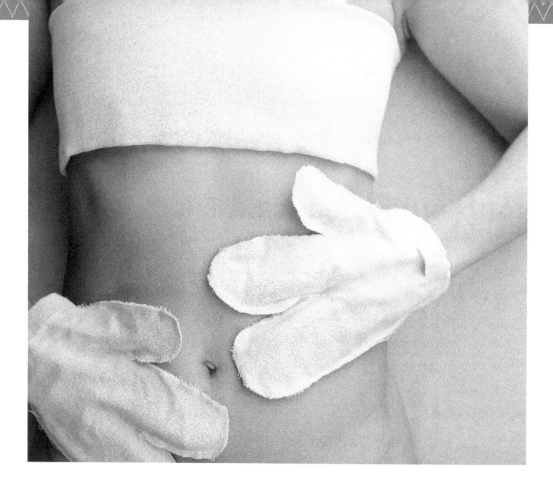

Daily Self-Care Practices

Stimulating, heating, lightening, and reducing are the characteristics that best describe the daily practices for the Mountain or those with a Mountain imbalance. Active and energizing breath practices, yoga poses, and exercise keep the abundant fluids of the body moving to assist cleansing. Massage with raw silk gloves, instead of or in addition to oil massage, improves the circulation and counters heaviness or stagnation.

Integrate these practices into your daily routine during the fourth week of the protocol and strive to continue them in everyday living. Make time for stimulating practices every few hours throughout the day, especially if your work requires you to sit and

be still for many hours. A five-minute break every few hours to move and breathe will help, but take a twenty-minute break if you can. Plan time in the morning for as many of these practices as possible to counter the heaviness at that time of day.

Raw Silk Massage

Garshana is the practice of dry massage with raw silk gloves. Much like dry brushing, the slightly rough and nubby texture of the raw silk exfoliates the skin, stimulates circulation and movement of lymph, and removes blockages to energy. The raw silk also creates a stimulating effect on the nervous system and has a lightening effect on the body. Follow the techniques for oil massage (see pages 70 to 74) while wearing the gloves and give yourself a dry, vigorous scrubbing each morning. If you have no coating on the tongue, you can apply one to two ounces of oil to your skin after the dry massage. If possible, follow oil application with dry heat or a hot shower or steam.

In the evening, give a short massage to the upper body. Use a dry, vigorous massage on the scalp with strong shampooing motions and use just enough oil on the fingertips to massage the face, neck, and shoulders without pulling on the skin. Bend over for this massage and rest your elbows on your thighs or knees to reduce tension in the shoulders. After the massage, use hot towels to compress the areas oiled—opening the pores, relaxing the muscles, and removing the excess oil.

Breathing Practices

The right nostril breath increases heat in the body. Use it in the morning to counter the cool qualities present or before meals to improve the strength of the digestive fire. The bellows breath is a stimulating practice that removes congestion from the lungs, increases energy, and has an overall effect of clearing the mind. Use it any time of day or night. Start each practice by finding a comfortable position to sit.

Right Nostril Breath

Block off the left nostril with one hand and continue deep belly breaths or the three-part breath (see page 75) for several minutes.

Bellows Breath

Take a few deep breaths into the belly. (If this is difficult, start with the deep belly breath and three-part breath on page 75.) Consciously inhale and exhale as fully and deeply as you can. Then speed up the rate of your breaths for thirty seconds without sacrificing their depth. The breath is like a bellows that you use to stoke a fire. Create an even breath in and out, increasing the pace so that you are breathing as fast as you can by the end of the one-minute practice.

After the last exhale, pause, keeping the breath expelled. Sit in stillness and notice how you feel. You may notice a calmness or clear mind. You may also notice that you have no need to inhale right away. You have so fully energized the body that it feels safe to relax. When you need to inhale, sip in a little breath and pause, holding the breath in without any strain. Wait until the body calls for more and enjoy the natural stillness between breaths. Breathe only as often and as much—or as little—as needed to feel comfortable for the next few minutes.

Exercise

Commit to daily vigorous cardiovascular exercise that induces sweating as your most important practice. Running, biking, hiking, swimming, skiing, jumping rope, and dancing are just a few of the possible options. For some, the duration required to induce sweating may be 15–20 minutes, but others may require 30 minutes or more. Find options that inspire and excite you so that this becomes a fun and permanent practice.

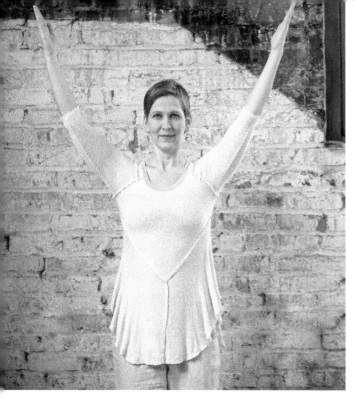

mountain with sun breath

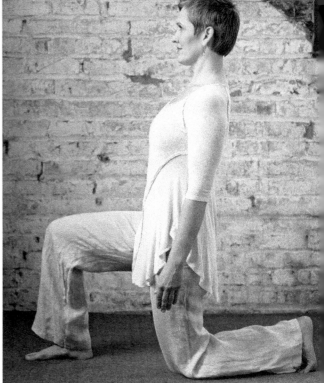

lunge

Yoga Poses

A balanced yoga practice should be stimulating, moving, warming, lightening, and energizing. It should include standing postures with long holds to build heat; back-bending postures to lighten and release the upper body; heating inversions, which require exertion; vinyasa or flowing movement; jumping; or shaking. Use the following postures together or separately when time is limited.

Caution: Unsupported or deep back bends and deep forward bends can place undue pressure on herniated or bulging discs or on the vertebrae when osteoporosis is present. To avoid this, focus on lengthening upward with a gentle lift of the heart instead of reaching backward in standing or unsupported backbends. Gentle, supported backbends are fine as long as there is no discomfort.

In forward bends, come forward with a flat back to avoid compression.

Forward bending with the head below the level of the heart is contraindicated for those with uncontrolled high blood pressure. To avoid this, bend forward only halfway so that the head and heart are equidistant from the floor.

Supported Backbend

Backbends open up the chest and the front of the shoulders, clear the channels for breathing, and lighten the body. Roll up a small towel and place it on the floor or your bed. Lie down so that your mid-back (bra line for women) arches over the towel. Relax in this position for several minutes while practicing deep full breaths.

Mountain with Sun Breath

Stand with your feet hip-width apart, toes spread wide, and the inside arch of the feet parallel to each other. Keep the knees slightly bent with the tailbone reaching downward to lengthen the low back area (this action also pulls the lower abdomen in toward the spine). Imagine holding a block or pillow between the upper thighs and give a gentle squeeze to hold it in place. From this position, lengthen the spine and reach upward through the top of your head.

Focus on your deep breath and move your arms overhead as you inhale, then return the arms to your side as you exhale. Continue with deep full breaths and coordinate the arm movements so that each movement takes the same amount of time as your breath. Now add a gentle backbend at the top of the inhalation (just enough to feel the heart area lift). When you exhale, bend forward with a flat back and reach toward the floor. Only come down as far as you can without rounding the spine—put your hands on your upper thighs for support. Inhale and stand up with a flat back, reaching up to Mountain position with your arms overhead at the top of the inhalation as you did before. Continue this until you feel heat building inside.

Warrior to Lunge

From the Mountain position, take one big step forward. Now bend both knees, drawing the back knee toward the floor. Straighten the back leg as much as possible: This is the Warrior position. Hold for one minute or longer, keeping your toes pointing forward and your torso upright. On an exhalation, bend the back leg, lowering the knee to the ground while keeping the front knee bent: This is a Lunge position. If you feel strong and steady, move between these two positions. Inhale when lifting up, and

exhale when coming down. Repeat several rounds and then switch legs.

Tips for Successful dietary Cleansing

These practices are appropriate for day-to-day maintenance for the individual with a Mountain constitution or imbalance. They are particularly important to follow during the fourth week of the protocol, but they must be modified for the final three days of digestive cleansing to avoid vigorous exercise, yoga, or breath practices.

Meals: Choose the amount of food and type of food for each meal based on your digestive fire. If you have coating on the tongue or a lack of appetite, choose lighter options such as soup or konji—or fast instead. Always eat your biggest or heaviest meal at lunchtime and make the other meals lighter. When possible, use the 100 Steps practice (see page 100) after meals. Drink a spicy tea 30 minutes before each meal and take nectar before or after the meal to improve your digestive fire. Always listen to your burp.

Snacks: Try not to snack between meals. Drink herbal tea or hot water if you feel hunger between meals, then snack on dried fruit or vegetable juice if necessary.

Water intake: Drink warm water with lemon upon rising, then sip on hot water or herbal tea throughout the day to improve the lymphatic circulation. Drink water at appropriate times so that it does not dull the digestive fire—one hour before or two hours after a meal.

Rest: Try to be in bed by 10:30 p.m. so that you can be asleep by 11 p.m. Sleep for only five to six hours; too much sleep can make a Mountain heavy and lethargic. If you are an early sleeper, rise at 4 a.m. for your morning practices. Avoid napping in the daytime and break up sedentary periods of the day with activity when possible.

Self-care: Prioritize the morning time for self-care, including as many practices as possible. Make vigorous exercise the most important practice in your day. If possible, try to stay warm and sweat every day. Avoid too much stillness and take breaks

100 STEPS FOR DIGESTION

To improve digestion, Dr. Vasant Lad, Founder of The Ayurvedic Institute, recommends a gentle walk of approximately one hundred steps after a meal. This practice could be done in conjunction with or in place of a digestive nap (see page 67). For the Mountain, this practice is better because napping in the daytime can increase heaviness.

Daily Schedule

5–6 a.m.	Wake, ideally after six hours of sleep.
	Drink warm water.
	Eliminate waste from the bowels and bladder.
	Do vigorous exercise, stimulating breath, and/or yoga poses.
	Clean the senses; observe the tongue.
	Do raw silk massage, potentially with a light layer of oil, and take a hot shower or sauna.
7:30 a.m.	Drink tea.
8 a.m.	Breakfast or fast, depending on your appetite.
10 or 11 a.m.	Self-care break with yoga poses or stimulating breath, followed by water intake.
Noon	Drink tea.
12:30 p.m.	Lunch, followed by 100 steps (see sidebar, above).
4 p.m.	Self-care break with yoga poses or stimulating breath, followed by water intake.
5:30 p.m.	Drink tea.
6 p.m.	Light dinner or konji, depending on your appetite.
9 p.m.	Drink warm water or tea if you are hungry (liquids only).
10 p.m.	Do a dry scalp massage, followed by a face, neck, and shoulder massage with light oil and a hot compress afterward.
10:30 p.m.	To prepare for bedtime, roll up a small towel and place it under your mid-back to create a supported backbend; rest for 10–15 minutes in this position; and go to sleep by 11 p.m.

throughout the day to practice stimulating and heating breath practices or yoga poses. Use oil on the body only when the tongue is free of excess coating.

Stress reduction: Use vigorous exercise, stimulating breath, and heating yoga poses to reduce stress.

"eat more" list
— for the mountain's daily diet and the lightening cleanse —

Choose foods that are **light, dry, and warm** and tastes that are **bitter, astringent, and pungent**.

Eat more of the following:

- **fruits** that are dried or astringent in taste, such as apples, apricots, berries, cherries, cranberries, figs, mangoes, peaches, pears, persimmons, pomegranates, prunes, raisins, and, in moderation, lemons

- **vegetables** that are bitter, astringent, or pungent, such as asparagus, artichokes, green beans, beets, bell peppers, broccoli, Brussels sprouts, burdock root, cabbage, carrots, cauliflower, celery, chili peppers, cilantro, corn, dandelion greens, daikon, eggplant, garlic, leafy greens, salad greens, onions, parsley, peas, potatoes (white, red, or gold), radishes, spinach, sprouts, winter squashes, turnips, and cooked tomatoes

- **grains** that are light, dry, or astringent, such as amaranth, barley, buckwheat, corn, granola, millet, quinoa, and rye

- **legumes** of all varieties

- **nuts and seeds** that are light, bitter, or astringent, such as pumpkin, flax, and sunflower seeds

- **condiments** that are pungent, such as basil, chili peppers, horseradish (wasabi), parsley, scallions, and, in moderation, seaweed

- **spices** in abundance, especially ones that are heating and astringent, such as black pepper, cinnamon, cayenne, cloves, garlic, ginger, hing, mustard seed, paprika, turmeric—and, in moderation, cardamom, coriander, cumin, and nutmeg

Use the following sparingly:

- **ghee** for cooking

- **sweeteners** such as honey or home-grown stevia (see sidebar on page 34)

- **oils** of corn, safflower, sunflower, or sesame

Limit or avoid foods that are heavy, dense, slimy, and oily; and tastes that are sweet, sour, and salty

LIGHTENING RECIPES

Most of the recipes are for warm, well-cooked foods and heating spices to kindle a dull digestive fire and improve digestion, assimilation, and elimination. The ingredients are light, dry, and heating, to counter excess Mountain qualities of heavy, moist, and cold. The spice mixes, teas, and recipes include a blend of calming and stimulating foods and spices, to keep circulation moving and counter stagnation while creating a calm but activated mind. Pungent, bitter, and astringent tastes also help the body break down old accumulations. These recipes can be part of a seasonal diet in the spring, year-round for those with a Mountain constitution or imbalance, or during the lightening dietary cleanse.

Cinnamon Millet Porridge With Apricot Cherry Sauce

During spring, the cold and moist qualities of the waning winter season have me wanting a warm, nourishing breakfast, but the melting accumulations inside me would rather I limit heavy, mucus-producing foods. Millet is a dry, astringent grain that can satisfy a strong appetite but leave you feeling light and energized. Warm, sweet cinnamon is also astringent and bitter, helping to dry up excess accumulations in the body as it aids digestion. The mildly sweet apricots and cherries make a tangy sauce for the porridge—no need to add sweetener.

YIELD • FOUR 1-CUP (235 ML) SERVINGS OF PORRIDGE; 1¼ CUPS (ABOUT 300 ML) SAUCE

1 quart (946 ml) water

1 cup (140 g) millet, uncooked

2 teaspoons Sweet Milk spice (see page 86) or 1 tablespoon Spiced honey (see page 86)

pinch of salt

squeeze of lemon

1 cup (246 ml) nut milk or grain milk

spiced honey, if more sweet is desired

For sauce:

1 cup (130 g) unsweetened, dried cherries (or fresh pitted cherries when available)

½ cup (70 g) dried apricots (or fresh pitted apricots when available)

1½ cups (355 ml) water

¼ teaspoon ground paprika

½ teaspoon (1 g) ground cinnamon

Place 3 cups (706 ml) water in a medium saucepan on high heat and bring to a boil. Add millet, Sweet Milk spice, salt, and lemon and stir together, then reduce heat to low and simmer for 20–25 minutes or until all of the water is absorbed. Place the cooked millet in a blender with the remaining one cup (240 ml) of water and milk, and carefully blend until creamy and smooth. The porridge should pour out of the blender; if not, add more water and blend again.

Caution: Leave the blender lid ajar or remove the center insert when blending hot items. The heat will create expansion and pressure inside the blender and could cause the lid to pop off while blending. You can also blend smaller portions to ensure your safety.

For the sauce: Combine all ingredients into a small saucepan and cook on medium heat for 15 minutes or until the fruits are mushy and most of the water has been absorbed. Transfer to a blender and mix on low until it makes a chunky sauce. For a thicker sauce, cook until all of the water is absorbed.

To serve, pour the porridge into bowls and place a few tablespoons of sauce on top, then gently swirl the two together. Serve with milk and spiced honey (see page 66) if more sweetness is desired.

Note: You can refrigerate the additional sauce or spread and use it another morning on porridge or grits. You can also use it like a chutney with kitchari. When made into a thicker spread, it is a perfect topping for a snack of Gingery Oatmeal Squares (see page 84).

Elevate Me Tea

Stimulating, bitter, spicy, and exotic, this tea will lift your senses with the smell, the taste, and the tingling it creates inside. Peppermint is a gentle digestive stimulant with a mild warming action that feels cool and tingly. It can relieve indigestion, gas, nausea, stomachache, headache, nervous tension, and insomnia. It can also lift or elevate the mind and emotions as it relieves tension in muscles. This is a great midday pick-me-up when your energy starts to dip!

YIELD · FOUR 1-CUP (235 ML) SERVINGS

1½ tablespoons (4.2 g) dried peppermint

1 tablespoon (8 g) ginger root, grated

2 teaspoons (1 g) dried nettles

1 star anise

1 quart (946 ml) hot water

Fresh mint to garnish

Combine all of the herbs in a large mesh strainer or tea ball and pour boiling water over the herbs into a thermos. Steep 10 minutes, remove the tea ball, and cover to retain the heat. To serve, pour into mugs and garnish with fresh mint leaves.

TIPS FOR YOUR TYPE

Fire: Drink in moderation.

Mountain: Reduce the ginger root to 1 teaspoon (2.7 g) and drink in moderation.

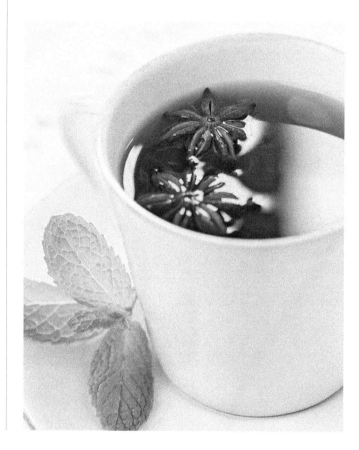

Roasted Poblano Stuffed with Chickpeas and Spinach

Chickpeas are one of the largest beans, with a slightly dry and rough texture. An abundance of heating and carminative spices can improve digestion and eliminate the production of gas that is common with these beans. Soaking the beans overnight—combined with a long, slow cooking process and the addition of kombu—will make them easier to digest. Enjoy the chickpeas alone as a stew or stuffed in a roasted poblano pepper with spinach.

YIELD • FOUR 1-CUP (129 G) SERVINGS OVER A ROASTED POBLANO PEPPER
WITH ¼ CUP (7.5 G) SPINACH

1 cup (170 g) chickpeas, soaked overnight

water, enough to cover chickpeas by 2 inches (5 cm)

2 strips of kombu

½ cup (75 g) chopped green bell pepper

½ cup (90 g) chopped tomatoes

¼ cup (60 ml) papaya juice

⅛ cup (30 ml) pomegranate juice

1 tablespoon (6 g) ground coriander

1 tablespoon (7.5 g) chili powder

2 bay leaves

1 teaspoon (1.8 g) ground ginger

½ teaspoon (1.2 g) ground cumin

½ teaspoon (2.3 g) black salt

½ teaspoon (1 g) ground black pepper

½ teaspoon (2.7 g) ground fenugreek

¼ teaspoon red pepper flakes

¼ teaspoon ground nutmeg

¼ teaspoon ground cinnamon

¼ teaspoon ground cardamom

To serve:

4 roasted poblano peppers

1 cup (30 g) spinach

Soak chickpeas overnight and discard the water in the morning. Place them in a large stockpot or pressure cooker with all of the ingredients for the chickpeas and then cover with at least 2 inches (5 cm) of water. Bring to a boil and then reduce heat and cover. When using a pressure cooker, secure the lid first and bring up to temperature, then reduce heat to low. Cook for 1–2 hours on low heat until the chickpeas are soft (less time in the pressure cooker). Remove the strips of kombu. (Their role was to add more nutrition and make the beans easier to digest, but they are a little too slimy for most palates.)

Cut the poblano peppers in half and remove the seeds. Place in an oven-safe baking dish and bake uncovered at 425°F (218°C) for 15–20 minutes or until the edges of the pepper brown without burning.

To serve: Place one pepper on a plate, cover with ¼ cup (7.5 g) spinach, and top with 1 cup (129 g) spiced chickpeas.

TIPS FOR YOUR TYPE

Breeze: Reduce chili powder to 1 teaspoon (2.5 g), eliminate red pepper flakes, and add 1 tablespoon (14 g) of ghee while cooking.

Fire: Reduce chili powder to 1 teaspoon (2.5 g) and eliminate ginger, black pepper, and red pepper flakes. Eat as a stew without the poblano pepper or over a bed of greens.

Savory Corn Grits with Spicy Kale

The foods of south Louisiana are pleasure to the senses—creamy, rich, and spicy—but they do not make for a trim waistline. I set out to make Cajun foods healthy with a little help from Ayurveda (and my Cajun husband). I added more bitter, green vegetables, used ghee instead of butter or lard, and incorporated lighter grains. It was a great success!

YIELD • FOUR 1-CUP (235 ML) SERVINGS

1 quart (946 ml) water

pinch of salt

1 cup (140 g) cornmeal

1 teaspoon (5 ml) sesame oil

1 teaspoon (2.6 g) chili powder

¼ teaspoon ground black pepper

¼ teaspoon ground cayenne pepper

For Spicy Kale:

2 cups (135 g) chopped kale

2 cups (135 g) chopped rainbow chard

½ cup (75 g) chopped bell pepper (yellow, orange, or red)

4 cloves garlic, peeled and finely chopped

1 teaspoon (2.7 g) ginger root, grated

1 teaspoon (5 ml) umeboshi vinegar or apple cider vinegar

1 teaspoon (5 ml) toasted sesame oil

¼ teaspoon ground paprika

¼ teaspoon ground black pepper

Place water and salt into a large 2-quart (2 L) saucepan or stockpot and bring to a boil on high heat. Slowly stir in the cornmeal and reduce heat to low. Continue cooking for 20–30 minutes, stirring every few minutes to avoid burning the bottom of the grits or creating firm chunks—the longer the cooking time, the softer and creamier the end result. In the last few minutes of cooking, add 1 teaspoon (5 ml) of sesame oil and all spices, including the nutritional yeast. Remove from heat and serve.

For the spicy kale, combine all ingredients with the remaining ½ teaspoon (2.5 ml) of sesame oil in a large skillet or wok and sauté, covered, for 8–10 minutes on medium heat until all of the water evaporates and the kale is wilted but not shapeless. Serve the corn grits like porridge in bowls and top with spicy kale.

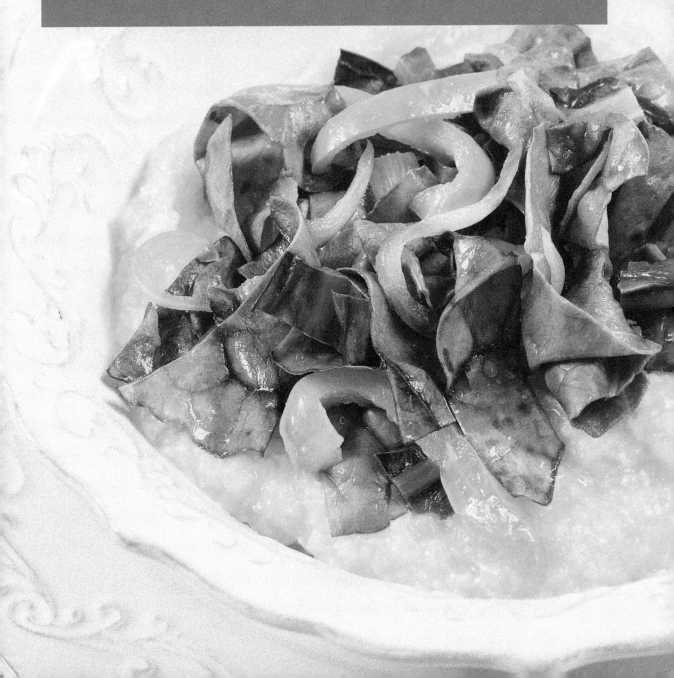

TIPS FOR YOUR TYPE

Breeze: For kitchari, add 1 tablespoon (14 g) ghee and use Warm the Breeze spice mix (see page 86) instead of the Lift the Mountain spice mix. For the Cajun veggies, do not use cayenne pepper, reduce garlic to one clove, and cook in 1 tablespoon (14 g) ghee. For chutney, replace the pepper with a pear. Eat amaranth occasionally, as it is very astringent and drying.

Fire: For kitchari, use 1 teaspoon (5 g) ghee and the Calm the Fire spice mix (see page 86) instead of Lift the Mountain spice mix. For the veggies, do not use garlic, peppers, onion, or cayenne. For the chutney, replace poblano with a pear and rosemary with 1 tablespoon (5 g) shredded coconut.

Amaranth Kitchari with Cajun Veggies and Cranberry Pepper Chutney

This version of kitchari is pungent and drying and will give the cool and moist qualities of the Mountain a gentle push toward balance. Amaranth is an astringent grain I like to use in the spring or whenever I feel heavy or congested. You can also use the one-pot cooking method to make this recipe, to improve digestion and reduce preparation time in the kitchen.

YIELD • FOUR 1-CUP SERVINGS KITCHARI AND VEGETABLES (221 G);
1½ CUPS (375 G) CHUTNEY

1 cup (184 g) split green mung beans, uncooked

1 cup (140 g) amaranth, uncooked

1 quart (946 ml) water

1 tablespoon (7 g) Lift the Mountain spice mix (see page 86)

For Cajun veggies:

½ cup (80 g) diced yellow onion

1 cup (120 g) diced celery

3 cloves of garlic, diced

¼ cup (25 g) chopped green onion

1 cup (90 g) chopped purple cabbage

1 cup (140 g) chopped turnips or rutabaga

1 cup (70 g) chopped collard greens

½ teaspoon (2.5 g) ghee or mustard oil

sprinkle of cayenne pepper

pinch of salt

For chutney:

½ cup (65 g) dried cranberries

½ cup (120 ml) water

½ poblano or Anaheim pepper, diced

1 date, soaked overnight in water and pitted

½ teaspoon (1.3 g) cumin seed

¼ teaspoon chopped rosemary

¼ teaspoon grapefruit zest

Rinse mung beans several times and pour off the water to clean any debris from the beans. Combine the beans, amaranth, and water in a large saucepan, then soak overnight. Cook the kitchari (mung beans and rice mixture) with Mountain spice mix on medium-low heat for 30–35 minutes or until the beans are soft and all of the water is absorbed.

Place all ingredients for the Cajun vegetables in a medium sauté pan and cook on medium heat for 25 minutes, stirring occasionally or until the cabbage and turnip/rutabaga are softened but still firm. Serve the vegetables over a bowl of kitchari with cranberry pepper chutney.

For chutney: Place all chutney ingredients except the grapefruit zest in a small saucepan and cook on medium-low until all of the water evaporates (approximately 10 minutes). Add grapefruit zest and transfer to a blender or food processor and mix on low for 30 seconds to 1 minute. The chutney will be blended but will still have some chunks.

Grilled Vegetables with Spring Bitters Salad and Sesame Garlic Dressing

The first precious little green plants that sprout in the spring are the perfect food-medicine Mother Nature provides to cleanse the body of accumulations from the winter season. These plants are bitter, astringent, and pungent in taste, and vary with climate and geography. Learning where and when to wild-harvest these plants can be a fun and exciting way to connect with nature, as well as with friends and family. In my experience, children love a "pick and eat" adventure hike and are quick to learn which plants to harvest. Look out for ramps, sorrel, nettles, fiddlehead ferns, garlic mustard greens, dandelion greens, and watercress in the wild—or plant radishes, peas, kale, spinach, or green onions in your garden.

YIELD • FOUR 1½-CUP (150 G) SERVINGS OF GRILLED VEGETABLES;
FOUR 1-CUP (36 G) SERVINGS OF SALAD GREENS; 1½ CUPS (311 G) DRESSING

one bundle of asparagus (approximately 30 thin stalks)

1½ cups (90 g) sweet pea pods

6–8 Spanish black radishes (160 g), thinly sliced

1 large red or orange bell pepper

1 teaspoon (5 ml) sesame oil

For salad:

½ ounce (10 g) dandelion greens

½ ounce (12 g) water cress

2 ounces (55 g) spinach

2 ounces (55 g) baby kale

2 tablespoons (12 g) chopped scallions or green onions

For dressing:

½ cup (72 g) sesame seeds, soaked

½ cup (72 g) sunflower seeds, soaked

1 tablespoon (8 g) grated or finely chopped turmeric root

1 tablespoon (10 g) grated or finely chopped garlic

½ cup (30 g) chopped parsley

1 large lemon, squeezed

1 tablespoon (15 ml) flaxseed or sesame oil

¼ teaspoon ground black pepper

¼ cup (60 ml) water

1 teaspoon (5 ml) liquid aminos

Coat the vegetables in a light layer of sesame oil and gently massage them by hand to evenly distribute the oil. Place on a cast-iron grill pan on medium-high heat or on an outdoor grill for a few minutes, until the vegetables soften and lightly brown along the grill lines. Turn the vegetables over and cook a few more minutes, then remove from the heat and let cool. Combine the washed and chopped salad greens in a large serving bowl and place the grilled vegetables over the greens. To serve, place 1 packed cup (36 g) of salad greens on a plate, cover with 1½ cups (150 g) of grilled vegetables, and top with 1–2 tablespoons (13–26 g) of dressing.

Note: You can also lightly steam the raw greens for easier digestion.

For dressing: Place all ingredients in blender
and puree on high until smooth.

Note: I like to make a larger batch of salad dressing and keep it refrigerated, so that I have a variety of flavors to choose from during the week.

Lighten Up Polenta with Squash Sauce

Cornmeal is dry and light in nature, so it is a natural choice for the Mountain, but it is often cooked with loads of butter, salt, and cheese or served with a heavy mushroom or tomato sauce. Sesame oil and spices add flavor in this recipe without excessive heaviness, and the sauce is made mostly of acorn squash, which has a slightly sweet yet bitter flavor. Served with broccoli rabe or other steamed green vegetables, this completes the palate of important tastes for the Mountain.

YIELD • SIX "PIE-SLICE" SERVINGS OF POLENTA; THREE CUPS (705 ML) OF SAUCE

1 quart (946 ml) water

pinch of salt

1 cup (140 g) cornmeal

1½ teaspoon (7.5 ml) sesame oil

1 teaspoon (2 g) chili powder

½ teaspoon ground black pepper

½ teaspoon ground paprika

¼ cup (14 g) nutritional yeast

For sauce:

1 medium onion, chopped

1 green pepper, deseeded and chopped

2 cups (115 g) seeded, peeled, and chopped acorn or butternut squash

1 cup (235 ml) water

1 large tomato

1 green chili pepper

1 tablespoon (2 g) Herbs de Provence

Serve with:

steamed or blanched broccoli rabe (or other green vegetables)

Place water and salt into a large 2-quart (2 L) saucepan or stockpot and bring to a boil on high heat. Slowly stir in the cornmeal and reduce heat to low. Continue cooking for 20 to 30 minutes, stirring every few minutes—the longer the cooking time, the softer and creamier the end result. In the last few minutes of cooking, add 1 teaspoon (5 ml) of sesame oil and all spices, including the nutritional yeast. Remove from heat and pour or spoon into a round pie plate to cool.

The polenta will firm up in 10–15 minutes and can be sliced into six pieces.

For the sauce: Sauté the onion and green pepper in the remaining ½ teaspoon sesame oil (2.5 ml) for 5–7 minutes on medium-low heat, then add the remaining ingredients and simmer for 20–30 minutes until all of the vegetables are soft and the sweet spicy smell fills the air. Transfer half of the sauce into a blender and puree, first on low and then on medium. Combine the chunks and the puree, then spoon the sauce over the polenta slices to serve.

Caution: Leave the blender lid ajar or remove the round center insert when blending hot items. The heat will create expansion and pressure inside the blender and could cause the lid to pop off while blending.

Note: To make a breakfast polenta cake, serve with the Apricot Cherry Sauce (see page 103).

TIPS FOR YOUR TYPE

Breeze: For the polenta, use half of the spices and 2 tablespoons (28 g) of ghee instead of sesame oil. Polenta is dry and rough in nature, so eat only occasionally. You can eat slices for breakfast with maple syrup or Banana-Berry-Delight Sauce (see page 84).

Fire: Prepare the polenta without any spices except nutritional yeast and salt—and use ghee instead of sesame oil. For the sauce and breakfast slices, see the Breeze recommendations above.

Spring Secrets Vegetable Chili

This chili is packed with many of my favorite spring secrets. The first is a small green daikon radish that has a slightly sweeter taste than the larger and more pungent white variety commonly sold in Asian markets. The watermelon radish looks just like a tiny watermelon when sliced, with a light green skin and a bright fuchsiacolored center; it also has a milder taste, similar to a white radish, that is not as sharp as a red radish. Burdock root is a bitter and pungent vegetable often used in cleansing teas. It is a long, straight, and sturdy brown root that has a carrot-like appearance and a white ringed center. Combined with the bright rainbowcolored stems of the leafy chard and the purple cauliflower, this dish is as beautiful as it is nutritious.

YIELD • SIX TO EIGHT 1-CUP (166–125 G) SERVINGS (DEPENDING ON COOKING TIME AND REMAINING LIQUID)

1 cup (250 g) black beans, soaked overnight

1 cup (170 g) pinto beans, soaked overnight

1½ quarts (1.5 L) water

1 piece kombu seaweed

¼ cup (30 g) chopped daikon or white radish

½ cup (30 g) chopped watermelon radish or rutabaga

1 cup (100 g) purple or white cauliflower

¼ cup (35 g) chopped burdock root or turnips

1 cup (67 g) chopped dandelion greens or rainbow chard

½ cup (80 g) chopped red onion

½ cup (75 g) chopped green bell pepper

3 cloves garlic, minced

1 jalapeño or hot pepper, finely chopped

1 teaspoon (2.6 g) chili powder

½ teaspoon (1.3 g) ground paprika

½ cup (30 g) chopped parsley, thyme, green onions, or a mixture of all three

1 teaspoon (5 ml) apple cider vinegar

¼ teaspoon salt

Soak the black and pinto beans in water overnight, then drain and combine with water and kombu. Cook on medium heat until boiling, then reduce heat to medium low and cover. Cook for 2 hours, stirring occasionally. Remove the kombu from the pot and add all remaining ingredients except salt. Continue cooking for another 25–30 minutes and add the salt in the last few minutes of cooking. The beans should be tender without any crunchiness, but the vegetables should retain their form and have a slight firmness. Beans vary in firmness based on their age and storage, so the amount of time necessary to make them tender always varies. If the beans are not done at this point, add another ½ to 1-cup (120–235 ml) water and continue cooking for another 15 minutes.

TIPS FOR YOUR TYPE

Breeze: Use sweeter vegetables like carrot and beet to replace the daikon and radish, 1 clove of garlic, and 15 sweet cherry tomatoes instead of a jalapeño or hot pepper.

Fire: Use carrots and broccoli to replace daikon and radish and cilantro instead of parsley mix. Omit garlic, jalapeño, and onion.

Tantalizing Tempeh and Stir-Fry Wrap

Tempeh is a fermented soy product that has a chewy texture. It is often marinated or covered with spices before cooking. It is simple to prepare quickly. I have a ceramic ginger grater that is easy to use and easy to clean. Just rub the ginger, turmeric, or garlic clove across the ceramic plate, then pour water over it to remove the pieces. Rinse with water again and it is clean. In less then two minutes your tempeh is prepared for cooking. The ceramic grater is also wonderful for fresh ginger tea or fresh grated spices like nutmeg or cinnamon.

YIELD • FOUR LARGE WRAPS OR SIX SMALLER WRAPS

10 ounces (283 g) tempeh, sliced into ½-inch-wide strips

1-inch by ½-inch (25 mm by 13 mm) piece ginger root, grated

1-inch by ½-inch (25 mm by 13 mm) piece turmeric root, grated

1 large clove garlic, peeled and grated

1 teaspoon (5 ml) toasted sesame oil

2 teaspoons (10 ml) liquid aminos

½ lemon, squeezed

For stir-fry:

1 golden beet, peeled and thinly sliced

1 black radish, thinly sliced

½ green bell pepper

10 Brussels sprouts, quartered

1 cup (100 g) chopped broccolini or Romanesco

3 ounces (84 g) baby spinach

¼ cup (60 g) water

For the wrap:

2 ounces (55 g) sprouts

gluten-free tortilla or wrap

hummus, optional

Place the sliced tempeh strips into a large sauté pan with the remaining ingredients on top of the tempeh. Lightly massage the ingredients into the tempeh with a hand or spoon (the turmeric may temporarily discolor your hand) and marinate 10 minutes. Cook on medium heat for 10 minutes, turning the tempeh frequently. Remove the tempeh and add the water and chopped veggies to the same pan to use the remaining spices. Cook another 10 minutes on medium heat, until the vegetables begin to soften but are still firm and crunchy in texture. Assemble the tempeh, stir-fry, and fresh ingredients in a gluten-free wrap or tortilla.

Optional: Use a prepared hummus to stick all of the ingredients in the wrap together—or make your own hummus.

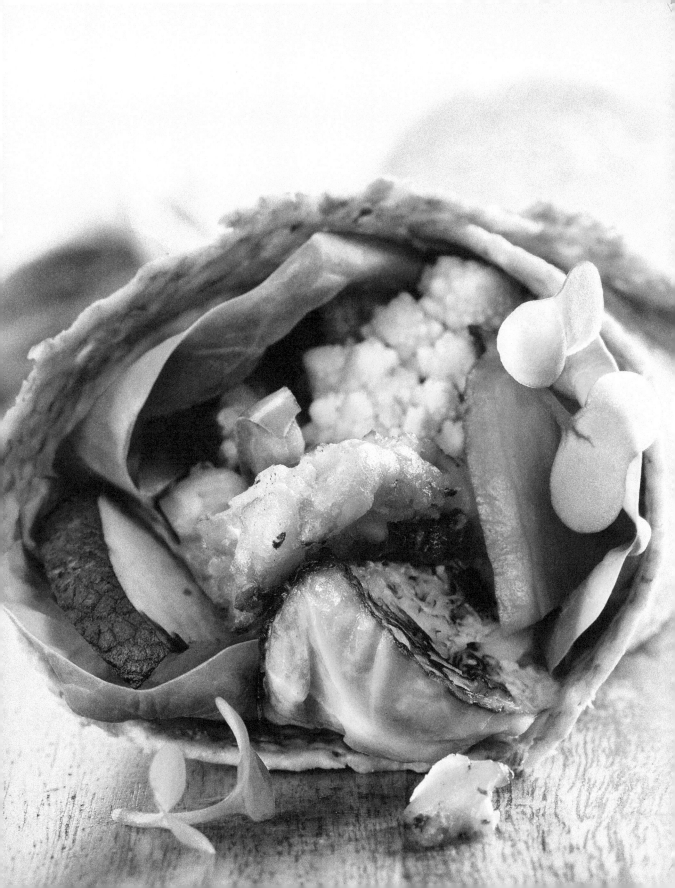

CHAPTER EIGHT

Cooling Cleanse & Diet

the purpose of this dietary cleanse is to lighten the body with a vegetarian diet of cooling foods and practices that reduce heat and accumulations. The diet consists of whole grains, legumes, nuts and seeds, fresh fruits and vegetables, cold-pressed oils and ghee, spices, and natural sweeteners that are all cooling in nature. These foods are predominantly sweet, bitter, and astringent in taste and are appropriate for those with a Fire constitution or imbalance.

These daily practices and self-care techniques are designed to be cooling, calming to the nervous system, and rejuvenating for the mind. The yoga poses, breathing practices, and exercise choices described aim to reduce Fire imbalances. Daily oil massage focuses on the head and feet and is applied with cooling oils in a gentle, soothing manner.

Daily Self-Care Practices

Actions for self-care of a Fire individual or a person with a Fire imbalance should be cooling, soothing, and calming. Avoid intensity or extremes. The Fire individual is commonly an "all or nothing" person with a strong drive for doing. Cultivating a middle-of-the-road mentality for this fourth week, and ideally for the rest of life, is important to finding balance.

Relaxing massage, breath practices, and yoga in the morning and evening will help set the tone for a day of activity and a night of sleep. Cooling practices in the daytime will counter the accumulation of heat from the season and climate, activity, or mental work. It is advisable to take some time away from a busy or intense work schedule during the week of cleansing or find a way to back off 30 percent from everything.

Oil Self-Massage

Daily self-massage can be done in the morning or in the evening, whichever time of day allows for more leisure in the massage (see pages 70 to 74 for instructions). If the full-body oil massage is in the morning, do a short head and foot massage at night before bedtime.

Breathing Practices

You can use the deep belly breath or three-part breath (see page 75) in the morning and evening to create relaxation, and the cooling breath during the daytime. It is helpful to take regular self-care breaks to practice this breath (followed by water intake) or to use it when emotions flare up. You can use both breath practices in a reclining or seated position.

Cooling Breath

Curl the sides of the tongue up to create a small channel and sip air in as if sipping through a straw. Feel the cool air move across the soft and hard palate as you inhale. This air passes across the tiny blood vessels that nourish the brain, relaying a cooling effect physically and emotionally. Exhale through the nostrils and continue this breath for several minutes or until you feel cooled and calmed.

Yoga Poses

Key words in a balancing yoga practice for a Fire individual are cooling, relaxing, surrendering, soothing, and gentle. An attitude of forgiveness and compassion for oneself and others is a good focus for yoga on and off the mat. Postures that open or wring out the middle region of the torso help release accumulated heat and toxins from the digestive organs. Twists, seated postures, cooling inversions, standing postures with wide legs, and forward bends are all appropriate. Childlike free-flowing movements are also helpful. Try these postures for their cooling effects.

Precautions: Inversions when the heart is higher than the head are contraindicated for individuals with uncontrolled high bold pressure; however an inversion of the legs (see right) with the head and the heart at the same level is fine.

Twists may cause undue strain on herniated or bulging discs in the spine, depending on the location of the injury. Use caution and move slowly so that you can stop if you feel pain or discomfort.

Twist

Sit in a comfortable position with both legs extended. Use cushions, folded blankets, or blocks under your hips so that you can sit without strain in the low back. Bend your left leg, cross it over your straight right leg, and place the sole of the foot on the floor near your right knee. Sit here and take deep belly breaths. Using your core strength, rotate your torso left and let your right hand rest on your left knee. Place your left hand behind you on the floor for support. Now breathe deeply and try to relax the belly and expand the rib cage. Stay here for several breaths and then slowly release. Switch legs and repeat.

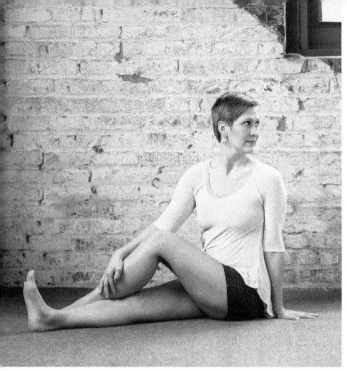

Twist

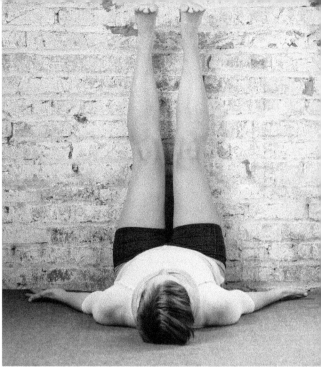

Inversion—legs up the wall

Inversion—Legs Up the Wall

Find a place along a wall where you can relax in a lying position with your straight legs extended toward the ceiling. Rest your legs on the wall and make yourself as comfortable as possible, with pillows or blankets for support. Cover the eyes and relax with deep belly breaths for 5–10 minutes. If you do not have a space along a wall, lie on the floor with knees bent at a 90-degree angle and rest your lower legs on a sofa or bed.

Exercise

Activities and exercise in nature are helpful for balancing the Fire individual. Nature itself has a calming effect on the Fire, and the cooling attributes of water enhance this. Swimming or walking near water is an ideal form of exercise, but any activity that is noncompetitive, leisurely, or playful is appropriate. To find balance, avoid exercise outdoors in the heat of the day and exercise that is intense or strenuous. Exercising in the cooler morning hours is advised.

Tips for Successful Dietary Cleansing

These suggestions are helpful on a daily basis for those with a Fire constitution or imbalance, but are an essential part of the fourth week of the protocol. For the final three days of digestive cleansing, modify these recommendations to avoid cold foods and exercise.

Meals: Drink cooling teas before or with a meal and take nectar with breakfast and dinner only (if your fire imbalance is strong, avoid nectar altogether). Eat enough food to be satiated and, whenever possible, take a digestive nap or use the 100 Steps practice after each meal.

Snacks: Snack on fresh fruit, vegetable juice, nut milks, or konji, but when hunger appears, always drink water; the desire for water is often mistaken as hunger.

Water: Drink warm water upon rising, then drink room temperature water throughout the day and avoid any drinks colder than that. Drink only a small amount of water with meals. Take self-care breaks to drink water between meals.

Rest: Try to be in bed without stimulation by 9:30 p.m., so that you can be asleep before 10 p.m. If a second wind arises, you may feel hungry and your sleep may be delayed. If hunger does arise, have a warm-milk drink, and if sleep is delayed, calm the nervous system with self-care practices.

Self-care: You can divide daily practices equally between morning and evening self-care routines. Calming practices should be the priority in the morning and evening and cooling practices during the day. You can do oil massage at any time, but you should do a head and foot massage every evening (even if you had a full-body oil massage in the morning).

Stress reduction: Spend time in nature, particularly around or in water for exercise and to reduce stress. Incorporate breath practices or yoga

Daily Schedule

6 a.m.	Wake, ideally after seven hours of sleep.
	Practice deep breaths.
	Practice twists (seated, as pictured on page 161, or lying in bed).
	Drink warm water.
	Eliminate wastes from the bowels and bladder.
	Walk in nature.
	Clean the senses; observe the tongue.
	Oil and shower.
7:30 a.m.	Drink tea or juice.
8 a.m.	Breakfast, followed by 100 steps if a nature walk did not happen earlier (see page 100).
10:30 or 11 a.m.	Self-care break with cooling breath or yoga poses, followed by water intake.
Noon	Drink juice or tea.
12:30 p.m.	Lunch (the biggest and heaviest meal), followed by 100-step walk or a digestive nap (see page 67).
4 p.m.	Self-care break, with cooling breaths, legs up the wall, and water intake.
5:30 p.m.	Drink tea or juice.
6 p.m.	Dinner.
9 p.m.	Practice deep breaths and candle-gazing meditation; oil head and feet, and place oil in ears.
9:30 p.m.	Prepare for bedtime; go to sleep by 10 p.m.

poses in your self-care breaks to diffuse intensity and heat during the day. Make time for stillness and avoid excessive work or stimulation during the fourth week.

"eat more" list
— for the fire's daily diet and the cooling cleanse —

Choose foods that are **cooling** in nature and tastes that are **sweet, bitter, and astringent**.

Eat more of the following:

- **fruits** that are sweet, cooling, or astringent, such as apples, avocadoes, dates, figs, grapes, limes, melons, pears, persimmons, pomegranates, raisins, and watermelon. Consume berries, cherries, oranges, peaches, plums, and pineapples only if they are sweet.
- **vegetables** that are green, bitter, and astringent, especially asparagus, broccoli, Brussels sprouts, celery, cucumber, green beans, green peppers, kale, leafy greens, lettuce, parsley, peas, yellow squash, zucchini, and all kinds of sprouts. *Eat in moderation*: carrots, cauliflower, cabbage, okra, potatoes, squash, and white or yellow onions (if well cooked). *Eat occasionally and in season*: fresh corn and fresh and sweet cherry tomatoes (from your garden, if possible)
- **grains** that are cooling or astringent, such as amaranth, barley, granola, basmati rice, wild rice, quinoa, oats, wheat
- **legumes** of all varieties, including tofu and tempeh
- **nut and seeds** that are cooling, such as coconut, almonds, sunflower, and pumpkin seeds
- **ghee and raw cow's milk** as a food-medicine for

lubrication and nourishment (If you consume dairy; otherwise use soy, almond, or cashew milk.)

- **oils** that are cooling, such as coconut, sunflower, safflower, and olive oil (all in moderation, because Fire individuals have a slightly oily quality by nature)
- **sweeteners** such as maple syrup, raw sugar, homemade stevia, or whole cane sugar
- **condiments** that are cooling, such as cilantro, lime, and mint; rock salt and seaweed in moderation
- **spices** that are cooling, sweet, bitter, or astringent, such as cardamom, coriander, cumin, fennel, saffron, turmeric; *eat occasionally*: cinnamon, fresh ginger, and nutmeg
- **mushroom broth, bone broths, or meat** of chicken, turkey, or venison (if you eat meat) for **non-cleansing** times or rejuvenation

Limit or avoid foods that are sour, salty, and pungent in taste, especially heating spices, hot peppers, garlic, uncooked onions, and vinegar.

COOLING RECIPES

The following recipes combine cooked and raw foods, with ingredients that are all calming in nature. Abundant green vegetables provide the bitter and astringent tastes that create a natural cleansing action in the body. All recipes involve mostly cooling ingredients, limiting salty, sour, and pungent foods and spices that increase the Fire imbalances. These recipes are good as part of a seasonal diet in the summer, for those with a Fire constitution or imbalance year-round, or as part of the Cooling dietary cleanse.

The Cool-Down "Iced" Tea

A tea made of coriander, cumin, and fennel is an Ayurvedic staple for aiding digestion without increasing the Fire, or heat, in the body. Cooled for summertime, this "iced tea" is better than traditional iced tea because it has no caffeine. Even though it is called "iced tea," serve it at room temperature so that it is easily digested and assimilated. Ayurveda recommends avoiding foods and liquids that are colder than room temperature. It is recommended that you drink the tea warm during the final three days of digestive cleansing.

YIELD • APPROXIMATELY 2 QUARTS (2 L) OF TEA; SIX 12 OUNCE (355 ML) SERVINGS

2 tablespoons (10 g) whole coriander seed

1 tablespoon (6 g) whole cumin seed

1 tablespoon (6 g) whole fennel seed

1–2 teaspoons (3.5–7 g) licorice root or 8 drops homemade liquid stevia

1 quart (946 ml) boiling water

4 cups (946 ml) ice, cubed or crushed

1 lemon, sliced for garnish

Place coriander, cumin, fennel, and licorice in a large mesh strainer or tea ball and place in a thermos. Pour boiling water into the thermos and allow the herbs to steep for 10–15 minutes, then transfer the tea to a pitcher, pouring it over ice to cool. Garnish each glass with a lemon slice to squeeze into the tea.

Caution: Anyone who has high blood pressure should not consume licorice root tea. Use homemade liquid stevia (see page 34) to add sweetness as an alternative.

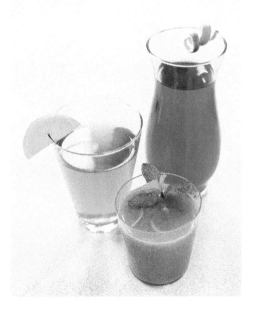

TIPS FOR YOUR TYPE

Breeze: Add 1 teaspoon (3 g) grated ginger to the tea.

Mountain: Add 1 tablespoon (8 g) grated ginger to the tea and use homemade liquid stevia sparingly.

The cool-down "iced" tea, summer soothe tea, cool as a cucumber summer cleanse juice (clockwise from left)

Turmeric "Latte"

Turmeric is a sweet and bitter root that is great replacement for the bitter of coffee. It can reduce inflammation, enhance proper functioning of the liver, cool the body, and clear out toxins. Warm turmeric milk is a common Ayurvedic recommendation for rejuvenation of the Fire imbalance. Turmeric's underlying effect on the body is calming (sattvic), so you can enjoy the ritual of your warm morning drink without the stimulating effects that bring craving and imbalance later in the day.

YIELD • TWO 1-CUP (235 ML) SERVINGS

2 cups (475 ml) fresh almond milk (see page 104)

½-inch by 1-inch piece (13 mm by 25 mm) turmeric root, grated

1 tablespoon (4 g) dried rose petals

1 teaspoon (1 g) dried chamomile flowers

pinch of nutmeg

pinch of cardamom

1 teaspoon (5 g) ghee

1 date, soaked overnight in water and pitted

Combine all ingredients except the date in a small saucepan and warm on medium-low heat for 10–15 minutes until the mixture comes to a gentle boil. Remove from heat, strain, and pour into the blender. Add the date and blend on low, then high, to create a foamy, frothy head on the milk. Pour into cups and serve.

Caution: Leave the blender lid ajar or remove the round center insert when blending hot items. The heat will create expansion and pressure inside the blender and could cause the lid to pop off while blending. You can also blend smaller portions to ensure your safety.

COFFEE

Regular consumption of bitter foods improves the flavor of the other five tastes. Bitter clears the palate and brings discernment to the tongue. Most people do not consume adequate bitter taste in the form of dark, leafy greens, nettles or bitter teas, bitter roots, or other green vegetables, so coffee with its roasted bitter flavor can easily feel like the antidote to that deficiency. Despite its delicious flavor, coffee is hot, sharp, and oily, and can increase these qualities in the body, dehydrate it, tax the liver, and overstimulate the digestive, elimination, and nervous systems.

TIPS FOR YOUR TYPE

Breeze: Add a pinch of ground ginger and an extra pinch of cardamom.

Mountain: Add ¼ teaspoon of ground ginger and cinnamon. Do not add rose, chamomile, ghee, or dates; sweeten as needed with spiced honey instead.

"Swami's Secret" Tofu Scramble

This recipe is dedicated to the swami who first introduced me to Ayurveda and Sanskrit, the language of traditional yogic and Ayurvedic texts. He excelled at storytelling, chanting, singing, cooking, and laughing. I still hear his deep, bellowing voice in my head every time I chant "Om." I am eternally grateful to him for his knowledge and for the culinary secret to making tofu scramble taste like eggs: "black salt." It is actually pink in color and very fine in texture, with a sulfur-like aroma—and is available at Indian markets. I also like to use nutritional yeast to add a "cheesy" flavor; it is full of B vitamins and ideal to consume with a vegetarian diet to ensure proper nutrition.

YIELD • FOUR 1-CUP (196 G) SERVINGS

15 ounces (420 g) firm tofu, pressed and crumbled

1 cup (71 g) chopped broccoli

1 cup (130 g) chopped carrots

1 cup (120 g) chopped yellow squash or zucchini

1 teaspoon (5 g) ghee or coconut oil

2 tablespoons (30 ml) water

1 tablespoon (15 ml) olive oil

½ teaspoon (1 g) ground cumin

½ teaspoon (1 g) ground fenugreek

½ teaspoon (1 g) ground coriander

1 teaspoon (2 g) ground turmeric

squeeze of lemon or lime

½ teaspoon (2 g) black salt (pink in color and very fine)

splash or capful of apple cider vinegar

1 teaspoon (1 g) nutritional yeast

For garnish:

1 tablespoon (3 g) chopped basil or cilantro

6–12 sweet cherry tomatoes (only when ripe and in season)

Drain the water from the tofu, slice it into ½-inch (13 mm) thick slabs, and "press" the tofu to remove the excess moisture. Place one clean cloth or towel over a cutting board and arrange the tofu on top of the towel. Then place a second cloth over the tofu and a heavy cookbook on top. Push down firmly and evenly on the cookbook to press the tofu for 1 minute, then leave the book in place for another 10 minutes.

Place the chopped veggies in a sauté pan with ghee or coconut oil and water. Cover with a lid and water-sauté for 15 minutes on medium heat. Push the vegetables to the sides of the pan, place the ghee or oil and spices in the center of the pan, and cook for 1 minute to release the aroma of the spices. Then crumble the slabs of tofu into the pan over the spices and stir together to coat the tofu evenly so that it turns an egg-like color. Add lemon or lime, black salt, and nutritional yeast directly to the tofu, stir gently, then mix in the other vegetables. Cook for a few more minutes to allow the flavors to meld. Garnish with chopped basil or cilantro and a few sweet cherry tomatoes only when fully ripe and in season.

Summer Sunrise Pudding

It is easy to see why chia is so popular. It is a high-protein food with a mild flavor that blends well with anything and has a slippery quality that is good for the digestive tract. This is one super food that is super easy to make into a healthy breakfast—and so delicious it could be dessert. My morning ritual in the summer starts with a sunrise at the beach and a bowl of fresh fruits, nuts, seeds, and coconut milk to keep me cool and nourished. If you don't have the beach, you can still have the sunrise in your bowl.

YIELD • FOUR 1-CUP (235 ML) SERVINGS

¾ cup (175 ml) coconut milk

¾ cup (175 ml) oat milk

¾ cup (102 g) sweet berries

1 mango, sliced

1 cup (115 g) granola (preferably with almonds and pumpkin seeds) or sprouted grains

¼ cup (48 g) chia seed

Fruits and fresh coconut for garnish

Combine coconut milk, oat milk, and ½ cup (75 g) fresh fruit in a blender and puree on high for 1 minute. Pour into a quart-sized (1 L) container with lid and mix in granola or sprouted grains and chia seed. Refrigerate overnight and serve in the morning topped with an assortment of berries, mango, or fresh coconut for garnish. You can also warm the pudding on low heat for a few minutes to counter the refrigerated cold.

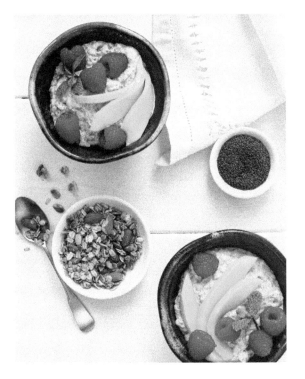

TIPS FOR YOUR TYPE

Breeze: Warm the pudding and eat in a warm season.

Mountain: This breakfast is very sweet, with cold and slippery qualities that are not good for the Mountain. Eat in small portions, only on occasion, and in a warm season.

Sweet Green Goodness Soup with Cucumber Raita

This soup is so creamy and sweet that I made it for my daughter as one of her first solid foods and for a friend receiving cancer treatment when nothing else was palatable. The recipe has had many variations throughout the years, but it remains a cooling, soothing staple for me. This version adds raita, a cooling side dish from traditional Indian cuisine, and a garnish of raw foods.

YIELD • FOUR 1-CUP (235 ML) SERVINGS

2 large zucchini, chopped into 1-inch (2.5 cm) cubes

½ cup (75 g) peas

1 large potatoes, chopped into 1-inch (2.5 cm) cubes

¼ cup (4 g) chopped cilantro, stems and leaves

¼ teaspoon (2 g) salt

1 cup (235 ml) water

1 teaspoon (5 g) ghee

½ lemon or lime, squeezed

For raita:

1 teaspoon (2 g) whole cumin seed

½ teaspoon (3 g) ghee

½ cup (115 g) unsweetened yogurt

½ cucumber, peeled and diced

1½ tablespoons (6 g) chopped dill

pinch of black pepper

pinch of mineral salt

For garnish:

5-10 zucchini strips, thinly sliced

pinch of sprouts (alfalfa, sunflower, mung, or pea shoots are all good choices)

1 teaspoon (2 g) ground pumpkin seeds

ADD IT!

For non-cleansing times, add ¼ cup (25 g) finely grated Parmesan cheese to the soup after blending and stir until melted.

Combine all ingredients in a medium stockpot, cover with a lid, and cook on medium heat for 20 minutes. At first, the solid chunks of vegetables will not be immersed in the water. Stir every 5 minutes, and as it cooks down, the vegetables will soften and sink into the water. The soup is done when all of the chunks are immersed in the water and soft. Transfer to a blender and puree. If you prefer chunky soup, puree half of the vegetables with all of the liquid and pour over the remaining chunks.

Caution: Leave the blender lid ajar or remove the round center insert when blending hot items. The heat will create expansion and pressure inside the blender and could cause the lid to pop off while blending. You can also blend smaller portions to ensure your safety.

For raita: Roast the cumin seeds with ghee in a small pan on medium heat for a few minutes until the seeds start to smell nutty and turn slightly brown. Remove from heat and spoon seeds into a blender with the yogurt, half of the cucumber, and the dill. Blend on low for 30 seconds, then transfer to a small bowl, mixing gently with the remaining cucumber, black pepper, and salt. To serve, pour a tablespoon of raita on each bowl of soup, then garnish with zucchini strips, sprouts, and ground pumpkin seeds.

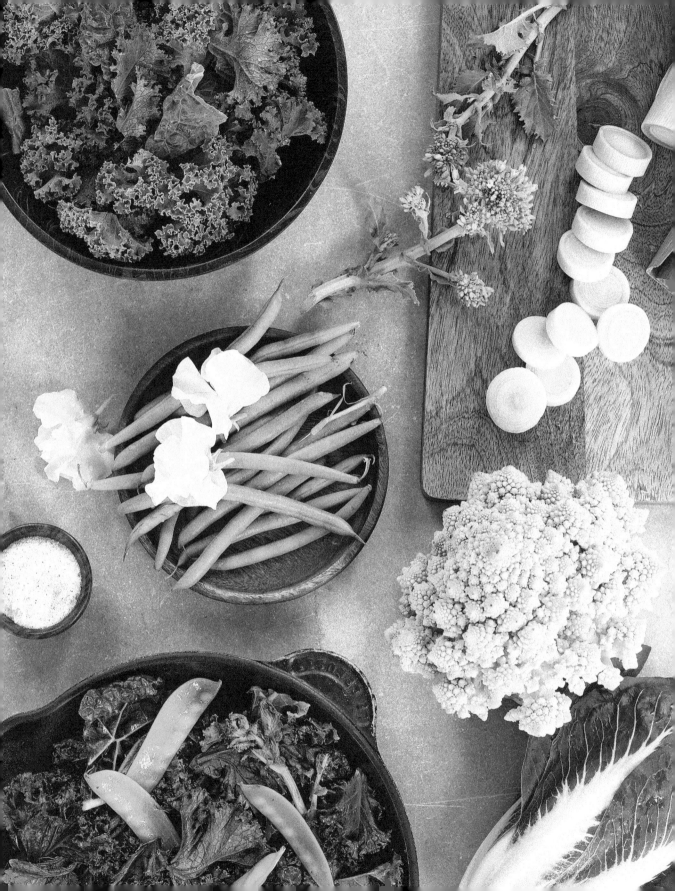

Green Beauty Sauté

In Ayurvedic consultations, I often tell clients who need a cooling diet to start by eating more green vegetables. This one tip will ensure that they eat more foods with the sweet and bitter tastes that are ideal for reducing heat. Most flower petals also have these two tastes, so any edible varieties are a beautiful complement to green salads or sautés. Many flowers and the essential oils extracted from them are used as remedies to open the heart and to clear heated emotions like anger or frustration. It is easy to be captured by the beauty of a flower and to sink into a moment of stillness in appreciation and awe. One simple way to include more awe-inspiring beauty in your food is by soaking broccoli or broccoli rabe in water and allowing it to blossom.

YIELD • FOUR 1½-CUP (170 G) SERVINGS

2 tablespoons (30 ml) water

1 teaspoon (5 ml) sunflower oil

1 cup (100 g) chopped Romanesco

½ cup (50 g) chopped leek

1 cup (71 g) flowering broccoli rabe

½ cup (35 g) chopped Treviso (bitter green variety of radicchio)

2 cups (135 g) chopped kale, three varieties

20 pea pods (60 g)

20 green beans (100 g)

1 teaspoon (5 ml) rose water or neroli (orange blossom) water, optional

pinch of mineral salt

For garnish:

sweet pea flowers or other edibles

mint or basil

In a large sauté pan or wok, combine all ingredients. Start with the water and oil, then place harder vegetables like Romanesco, leek, and broccoli rabe in the pan and layer on top the lighter, softer, or leafy vegetables. Cover and cook on medium heat for 5–10 minutes so that the harder vegetables are lightly crunchy and the leafy vegetables start to wilt. Sprinkle the rose or neroli water and salt over the vegetables and then remove from heat. Garnish with edible flowers, mint, or basil and serve.

TIPS FOR YOUR TYPE

Breeze: Include more of the sweeter green vegetables like pea pods and green beans and reduce the amount of strong bitters like Treviso. Cook a few minutes longer to ensure that the harder vegetables are soft, and cook in ghee instead of sunflower oil.

Mountain: Steam vegetables and sprinkle black pepper on top.

NOTE

You can aid digestion of raw foods with a small amount of heating foods or spices. The right amount of heat for each person varies, and some Fire individuals will not be able to tolerate any heating foods. Modify as needed to make sure you do not feel any discomfort or heat sensations in the stomach after a meal. In this recipe, the bell peppers are sweet and juicy but have a mild heating nature; apple cider vinegar is sour but used in small amounts; and scallions are heating, parsley slightly less heating, and mint cooling. Choose the mix of ingredients that works for you.

TIPS FOR YOUR TYPE

Breeze: Raw foods are hard to digest, so use softer, sweeter lettuce varieties and eat only in a warm season. Alternately, eliminate the cucumbers, choose baby kale greens, and lightly sauté all ingredients with the hijiki. Use umeboshi vinegar instead of apple cider vinegar in the dressing.

Mountain: Eliminate cucumbers, choose baby kale greens, add ½ jalepeño pepper (diced), and lightly sauté all ingredients with the hijiki. For the dressing, add ¼ teaspoon grated ginger and a sprinkle of black pepper and add an extra ¼ cup (60 ml) of water to make it thinner.

Hijiki Rainbow Salad with Avocado Pumpkin-Seed Dressing

Seaweed is a nutrient-packed, mineral-rich food that can bring the perfect amount of salt to the Fire's diet. You can choose from many varieties of seaweed; some can be cooked with foods to improve digestion or flavor and others are eaten dried or rehydrated. I cook kombu with beans to improve digestion and reduce gas. Dulse is great dried and chopped into small pieces to sprinkle on salads or soups. Nori is a perfect healthy snack, toasted in the oven with a little oil and rock salt. Hijiki comes dry and needs to be rehydrated before eating, but it can be eaten raw or cooked to add more flavor. This recipe is inspired by a salad I have enjoyed at my favorite sushi restaurant, Bizen, in Western Massachusetts. I have added more sweetness with golden raisins and jicama, a root with the light and crunchy texture of a water chestnut and an apple-like flavor.

YIELD • FOUR TO SIX 1-CUP (200–133 G) SERVINGS DEPENDING ON THE VOLUME OF THE LETTUCE VARIETY

12–16 ounces (340–455 g) of leafy greens, like frisée, green or red leaf lettuce, or baby kale

3 small bell peppers, julienned

¼ small jicama, sliced into matchsticks or grated

1 small carrot, sliced into matchsticks or grated

½ cucumber, peeled and sliced into matchsticks

¼ cup (34 g) golden raisins

¼ cup (6 g) dry hijiki, soaked

1 teaspoon (5 ml) olive oil

squeeze of lemon or lime

sprinkle of maple syrup

For dressing:

¼ cup (36 g) pumpkin seeds, soaked

⅛ to ¼ cup (30–60 ml) water

1 ripe avocado

1 tablespoon (15 ml) apple cider vinegar

⅛ cup (8 g) chopped parsley, mint, or scallions

1 tablespoon (15 ml) sunflower oil

Wash and place leafy salad greens in a large salad serving bowl and arrange chopped vegetables and raisins on top of the greens. Rehydrate hijiki in a bowl of water for 10 minutes, then drain and place in a small sauté pan with oil, lemon or lime, and maple syrup. Cook on low for 15 minutes to tenderize the seaweed and allow the flavors to be absorbed. Place the hijiki in a mound in the center of the greens and serve with dressing.

For dressing: Soak pumpkin seeds for several hours in a cup of water, then drain and place in a blender with all other ingredients. Blend on low, then on high for a few minutes to make a creamy pourable dressing. More water will make it thinner and easier to spread evenly on the salad.

Warm Slaw

Cold and raw foods should be reserved primarily for a hot season when there is a strong need for cooling the internal environment of the body. If you want to enjoy the flavor and texture of raw vegetables in a cooler season or climate, here is a new twist on traditional coleslaw. The vegetables are grated or finely chopped and then lightly water-sautéed to retain the color, fresh flavor, and texture without the cold. Sunflower oil and avocado replace the heavy mayonnaise sauce of traditional coleslaw with good healthy fats.

YIELD • FOUR 1-CUP (139 G) SERVINGS

1 cup (110 g) finely chopped or grated carrots

1 cup (70 g) finely chopped or grated purple cabbage

1 cup (120 g) finely chopped or grated celery root (celeriac)

1 cup (70 g) finely chopped kale

2 tablespoons (30 ml) water

2 tablespoons (30 ml) sunflower oil

¼ cup (16 g) minced dill

pinch of mineral salt

1 lime, squeezed

1 ripe avocado, sliced

Combine the chopped carrots, cabbage, celery root, and kale in a sauté pan with the water and a splash of sunflower oil. Sauté, covered, on medium heat for 4–7 minutes. A shorter cooking time will retain the firm texture of the vegetables, while a longer time will make them softer and easier to digest. Remove from heat and add the remaining sunflower oil, dill, salt, and lime juice, then mix thoroughly. Add sliced avocado for garnish.

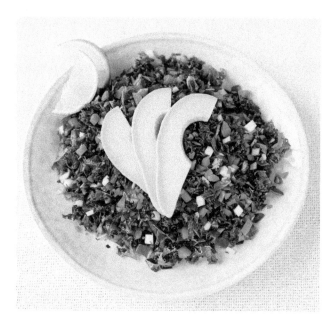

TIPS FOR YOUR TYPE

Breeze: Use sesame oil cooked with a little chopped garlic, add chopped chives, and cook longer.

Mountain: Use sesame oil cooked with 1 clove garlic, 1 chilli pepper, and chives (all chopped) and cook for a moderate amount of time. Omit avocado.

CHAPTER NINE

Taking it Deeper: Traditional Ayurvedic Cleansing

In the daily practices of Ayurveda, the main goal is pacifying the doshas so that they are not creating problems or imbalances in the body. The excess doshas accumulate over time and at some point pacification is not enough; the doshas need to be removed. Daily and seasonal self-care practices that focus on prevention only pacify the doshas, but when health is lost, Ayurveda recommends an intensive system of cleansing and rejuvenation, called panchakarma, to eliminate excess doshas along with environmental toxins and accumulated ama. For our purposes, this practice is called eliminatory cleansing.

Panchakarma Retreats

Panchakarma refers to the five (pancha) actions (karmas) used to cleanse accumulated doshas and ama from the body. These five actions are *vamana* (emesis or therapeutic vomiting), *virechana* (purgation from castor oil or herbal formulas), *niruha basti* (herbalized enema, sometimes called cleansing enemas), *nasya* (herbal oils or dry herbs administered through the nostrils), and *anuvasana basti* (oil enema, sometimes called nourishing enemas). Sometimes *rakta moksha*, or mild blood-letting, is named as the fifth action, instead of anuvasana basti, but that is not as common a practice. It is also not to be compared with the very depleting and excessive use of blood-letting that has historically been used, often to great detriment.

When people discuss the panchakarma process, however, they are usually referring not only to these five cleansing actions but also the preparatory and post-panchakarma stages of a comprehensive cleanse. This comprehensive cleanse includes preparing the body to receive the five actions safely and effectively, undergoing one or more of the five actions, supporting the body to stabilize afterward, and, finally, rejuvenating the body and mind. Traditionally, it is a process that takes a minimum of one month but often several months to complete.

In India, a patient would stay at a hospital or clinic for the entire length of the process and be completely isolated from stressors of life with little or no contact with the outside world. Panchakarma would be completed under the direct supervision of an Ayurvedic doctor, or *vaidya*, and patients would be cared for with daily massage treatments, oils, herbs, food, and rest recommended specifically for their particular imbalance. The ultimate goal of this process was full and complete rejuvenation of all of the bodily tissues, the senses, the mind, and emotions. It was reported to rejuvenate even bone, teeth, and hair of elderly individuals, adding thirty to forty years to their life span.

Although it is still possible to receive this traditional treatment in some places in India, most modern-day panchakarma programs, especially in the West, have been modified to make them more accessible. First, they are designed to allow the client to stay at home for most of the process. This limits the residential time in the personal care of the vaidya. In this way clients can reduce their time away from home and daily life to one or two weeks, making it more accessible to most people. This, however, does make the experience much different and less intense and comprehensive than the traditional system allows. It also places the client in the position of taking personal responsibility for carrying out most of the preparations before and rejuvenation after cleansing without direct supervision.

The Four Stages of Panchakarma

The traditional comprehensive cleanse that we usually refer to as panchakarma has four stages. *Ama-pachana*, the first stage, involves practices to burn up ama in the digestive tract, remove congestion and blockages in the channels, and strengthen the digestive fire.

Traditionally, recommended practices would include warm oil massage treatments, very gentle yoga postures or breathing practices to increase the strength of the digestive fire, a simple diet with little to no oil or salt, and herbal teas or medicinal formulas that are pungent, bitter, or astringent in nature. In nonresidential preparations, recommendations usually involve dietary changes, daily cleansing practices, and herbal intake. These practices serve to clear the digestive tract before the second stage, so that the ingested ghee does not create more congestion.

Stage two aims to lubricate the digestive tract and soften the tissues. This is accomplished internally with ingestion of ghee and externally with the application of oil and heat. Oleation, or application of oil (*snehana*, see sidebar on right), and sudation, application of heat (*swedana*), are the two main therapies used to move the accumulated doshas from their locations around the body back to their homesites. The purpose of this stage is to soften the tissues, open subtle channels of the body, and create a clear pathway for old stored toxins and accumulated doshas to return to the digestive tract for elimination from the body through the five actions. The cleansing actions to remove the excess doshas cannot be carried out safely unless the oleation process is done properly. The goal is to saturate the tissues thoroughly from the inside and the outside.

In the third stage, each of the five actions of panchakarma is used to remove one or more of the accumulated doshas. Not all clients need all of the actions. Some clients may need only one action, while others may need several. *Bastis*, or enemas, remove excess vata dosha. Purgation with castor oil or other herbal formulas removes excess pitta dosha. Therapeutic vomiting, or vamana, removes excess kapha dosha. Mild blood-letting, or rakta moksha, removes excess pitta, and nasya, or therapies applied through the nostrils, removes accumulated doshas from the brain, nervous system, or the mind. Even today, blood-letting is often performed with leeches for obstinate skin diseases or stubborn, chronic, localized pain. The leeches are usually applied near the area of the skin eruption or the area of pain, to draw fresh blood through the problem area. Rakta moksha is rarely practiced in the West, though some vaidyas may recommend that certain individuals with high pitta donate blood.

The deepest part of the cleansing process is carried out during the third stage, but the cleansing does not stop there. In fact, the actions of panchakarma really just open the flood gates, so that the body can continue the cleansing process for the next few months. It is very important to understand that this final phase of rejuvenation is just as important as any other stage.

The body is in a vulnerable state at this point in the process, because the excess doshas that were eliminated may have been accumulating for decades and the body has compensated for these imbalances. Imagine pulling a weed up out of the ground and observing the space in the soil the roots occupied. This empty space in the soil is much like the empty space in the body after the excess doshas have been removed. It takes time and proper care to rebuild

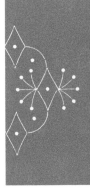

OLEATION

Picture a twig on a tree—it is soft, green, flexible, and full of sap. It does not break easily. This is the state of our human bodies as children—soft, juicy, and flexible. Like a twig that has fallen off the tree, we become drier and more brittle with age. Now imagine taking that dry twig, soaking it in warm oil, and steaming it. The oil will penetrate into the small channels or openings and saturate it. Eventually, the twig will be flexible enough to bend and twist again without breaking. This is the goal of oleation in panchakarma.

healthy, strong, balanced tissues to fill the weak spaces. Rejuvenation, the fourth stage, takes one to three months to complete. Ayurvedic doctors often recommend that patients care for themselves during this period as if they have just had surgery.

The rejuvenation period consists of daily self-care practices, diet, herbal preparations, and lifestyle recommendations tailored to each individual to rebuild healthy tissues and prevent future accumulation of the imbalanced doshas. The diet only gradually becomes heavier and more nourishing than during the cleansing process, and herbal formulas are often sweet and building in nature. Daily oil massage with specific oils is recommended, as well as the daily routine of cleansing practices for the organs of elimination and the senses (dinacharya). Yoga, breathing practices, exercise, and rest are prescribed in proper amounts for rejuvenation.

The Ghee Cleanse

When panchakarma is not possible—due to time constraints, finances, or other factors—but a deeper cleanse is required, some Ayurvedic practitioners will suggest a ghee cleanse. These individually tailored practices take several forms, but the common link is using ghee to cleanse (similar to the second phase of panchakarma). Just as in panchakarma, this practice requires guidance by a professional. Some practitioners call it a "home panchakarma," as Dr. Vasant Lad describes in the book *Ayurvedic Home Remedies*, while other practitioners incorporate it with other cleansing practices, as Dr. John Douillard does in his book *Colorado Cleanse*. These are modern adaptations not mentioned in the classic texts.

Ghee cleanses typically involve burning up ama and toxins in the digestive tract, and this is accomplished through eating a lightening diet similar to the

WHY CLEANSE WITH GHEE?

Ayurveda considers ghee the best food-medicine. It lubricates the mucosae of the digestive tract, helps regulate digestion and hormones, lubricates the joints, and can increase good cholesterol. It can penetrate into minute channels of the body, opening and clearing them to restore proper flow of oxygen, nutrients, and waste products.

Our guiding intelligence will store toxins or impurities away from the circulation and flow of daily metabolic activities. The storage site of choice is our adipose tissue, or fat. Even on a cellular level, toxins are stored in and transported by fat molecules. The cell membrane is permeable by fat, so it makes sense that to cleanse the body of unwanted wastes, a lipophilic, or fat-loving, substance would be the ideal carrier. Ghee is that ideal carrier.

final days of your month-long protocol and taking pungent, bitter, or astringent herbs and teas. Then ghee is ingested in increasing amounts for a period of four to seven days, during which kitchari is the recommended mono diet. A daily self-massage with warm oils is followed by application of heat for all or some of the cleansing days.

After the oleation is complete, castor oil or other purgatives are administered to release the contents of the digestive tract and eliminate the excess doshas that have returned to their homesites from the process of oleation. One or more days of rest is recommended for rejuvenation, along with an oil enema to nourish and soothe the colon.

The ghee cleanse is appropriate for those who have adequate strength to undergo the purgation process, because, like panchakarma, it not only removes ama and toxins (as many modern cleanses do), but also goes a step further to remove the excess doshas. This is a deeper cleanse and requires more strength to complete without creating imbalance.

Partnering with an Ayurvedic Professional

It is a goal of Ayurveda to empower individuals to take responsibility for their own health and use the tools of self-awareness and practices of self-care to create balance. Still, it is also a good idea to have an experienced guide along the way, particularly in cases when imbalance has already progressed through the six stages to a fully manifested disease.

Improper practices of cleansing can drive the doshas and toxins deeper into the body and create more imbalance. Only experienced Ayurvedic doctors are qualified to advise patients on the state of health for maintenance and the state of disease. They can navigate the challenging and complicated world of allopathic medicine and pharmaceutical drugs and weave its approaches masterfully with the herbal remedies and natural practices of Ayurveda. For deep cleansing, this guidance is essential: Panchakarma should never be done without an Ayurvedic doctor or an experienced practitioner.

An Ayurvedic practitioner or lifestyle consultant who is not trained specifically in panchakarma practices can still advise about practices for maintaining health and balancing the doshas when they have become aggravated. An Ayurvedic professional can recommend food-medicines and spices as well as daily self-care practices, yoga poses, breathing practices, lifestyle changes, Ayurvedic bodywork therapies, and daily, dietary, or digestive cleansing practices. Truly, the simple basics of Ayurveda are so powerful when practiced regularly that these can often bring about life-changing improvements.

Appendix

Constitution Checklist

— courtesy of banyan botanicals, created by dr. claudia welch —

Place a check mark next to each statement that has applied to you throughout your life. Total the number of checks in each category to determine your predominance.

_ My lifelong tendency has been to be thin and lanky.

_ I find having a routine in life challenging.

_ My skin tends to be rough and dry, even if I don't live in a dry, arid climate (and especially if I do).

_ My joints are fairly prominent.

_ My teeth are protruded and/or crooked.

_ My hair is kinky, curly, and tends to be dry or frizzy.

_ It is usually easy for me to lose weight and I usually have difficulty gaining weight.

_ I usually enjoy hot weather.

_ I tend to dislike wind.

_ I tend to dislike very dry climates.

Total Breeze/vata characteristics: _____

_ I have a medium build with medium bone structure.

_ I enjoy competitive activities and enjoy physical or intellectual challenges.

_ My teeth are medium-sized and/or a little yellow (stained doesn't count).

_ I have fair skin that sunburns easily.

_ I have a lot of moles or freckles.

_ I am or am becoming bald, I have grayed early, or I have thin or fine hair.

_ My eyes are sensitive to light.

_ I prefer a cool climate to a warm one.

_ I dislike heat, especially humid heat, and feel easily fatigued by it.

_ I have a sharp, intelligent, aggressive mind.

Total Fire/pitta characteristics: _____

_ I have a sturdy constitution with a large bone structure.

_ I have had a lifelong tendency to always be at least a little overweight.

_ My teeth are naturally large, straight, and white.

_ My hair is thick and lustrous.

_ My eyes are large with long, full, luxurious lashes.

_ If given the opportunity, I can easily sleep deeply for 8–10 hours per night.

_ I gain weight easily and have difficulty losing weight.

_ My facial features are rounded, with full, moist lips.

_ I tolerate most climates well, but have usually preferred hot, dry weather.

_ My energy and stamina are consistent. When I have a lot to do, I do it at a pace that I can maintain for a long time.

Total Mountain/kapha characteristics: _____

Imbalance Checklist

— courtesy of banyan botanicals, created by dr. claudia welch —

Place a check mark next to each statement that applies to you at this time. Total the number of checks in each category to find your predominant imbalance.

_ I have been feeling nervous, fearful, panicky, anxious, or frantic.

_ I have twitches, tics, tremors, or spasms in my body and I fidget a lot.

_ My skin is dry and easily chapped.

_ I have been suffering from dry, hard stools, constipation, gas, or bloating, or I have been having loose stools due to emotional upset.

_ I feel I am underweight.

_ Lately I have a stronger dislike of the wind and cold than usual.

_ I have a difficult time tolerating loud noise.

_ My sleep has been light, interrupted, restless, or disturbed.

_ I feel scattered, spacey, and have difficulty concentrating or have poor memory.

_ I am prone to overthinking or worrying.

Total Breeze/vata imbalances: _____

_ I have a red, inflamed, or burning rash; acne, cold sores, or fever blisters.

_ There is acute inflammation in my body or joints.

_ I have acid reflux, heartburn, acid indigestion, or a gastric or peptic ulcer—or a tight, burning feeling in my stomach or digestive tract.

_ I feel nauseated or uncomfortable if I miss a meal.

_ I have been having loose stools that are not due to emotional upset.

_ I have been feeling uncomfortably warm or hot.

_ I have been feeling frustrated, irritable, or angry.

_ I can be easily judgmental, impatient, critical, or intolerant of others.

_ My eyes have been red, bloodshot, inflamed, or sensitive to light.

_ I expect perfection of myself or others.

Total Fire/pitta imbalances: _____

_ I have excess mucus in my body or nasal passages or lung congestion.

_ I have a thick, white coating on my tongue.

_ My bowel movements are slow, sticky, sluggish, or feel incomplete.

_ I am overweight.

_ It is difficult for me to wake up in the mornings, even if I sleep deeply for 8–10 hours, and I feel lethargic throughout the day.

_ I have been feeling slow, foggy, dull, lethargic, or heavy.

_ In the morning I have to cough up a lot of mucus.

_ I have a deep, wet cough that produces a lot of mucus.

_ I feel complacent, stubborn, and resistant to any change—or my close friends and family tell me that I am very slow to change or to make a decision.

_ I am prone to excessive emotional eating, especially of sweet, heavy foods.

Total Mountain/kapha imbalances: _____

Cleansing Table

When picking a cleanse, you should choose one to correct your predominant imbalance. If, after taking the Constitution and Imbalance Questionnaires, you have more than one predominant imbalance, refer to the table below to determine which cleanse is right for you. If you are balanced, then you should pick your cleanse based your constitution, with mindful consideration of the season.

Using the Table

Step 1 Find your constitution in the far left column.

Step 2 Move across the chart to find your predominant imbalances and use the key below to determine which cleanse is appropriate (G, C, or L) and if you need modifications (*b, *f, *m, in cold, in hot, or in particular seasons).

Possible Imbalances:

BF: equally predominant Breeze and Fire imbalances

BM: equally predominant Breeze and Mountain imbalances

FM: equally predominant Fire and Mountain imbalances

BFM: Breeze, Fire, and Mountain imbalances equally

Key to Cleanse Options:

G: Grounding

C: Cooling

L: Lightening

Key to Modification Options:

*b: Use the Breeze modifications.

*f: Use the Fire modifications.

*m: Use the Mountain modifications.

in cold: Use in a cold or cool season.

in hot: Use in a hot or warm season.

Cleansing Table

CONSTITUTION	IDEAL SEASON	BF IMBALANCES	BM IMBALANCES	FM IMBALANCES	BFM IMBALANCES
BREEZE	Autumn	G in cold/C in hot	G or L*b	C in hot/ L in cold	G
BREEZE-FIRE	Between summer/ autumn	G in cold/ C in hot	G or L*b	C in hot/ L in cold	G
BREEZE-MOUNTAIN	Autumn + spring	G in cold/ C in hot	G in autumn/ L*b in summer/ L in spring	C in hot/ L in cold	G or L*b
FIRE	Beginning and end of summer	G in cold/ C in hot	G in autumn/ L other times	C in hot/ L*f in cold	C
FIRE-BREEZE	Between summer/ autumn	G in cold/ C in hot	G in autumn/ G*m in summer/ L in spring	C in hot/ L*f in cold	C in hot/ G in cold
FIRE-MOUNTAIN	Between spring/ summer	G in cold/ C in hot	G in autumn/ L other times	C*m in hot/ L*f in cold	C in hot/ L*f other
MOUNTAIN	Early spring	G in cold/ C in hot	G in autumn/ L other times	C in hot/ L other	L
MOUNTAIN-BREEZE	Spring + autumn	G in cold/ C in hot	G*m or L	C in hot/ L other	L or L*b
MOUNTAIN-FIRE	Between spring/ summer	G in cold/ C in hot	G*m or L	C*m in hot/ L*f in cold	L*f in cold/ C*m in hot
BREEZE-FIRE-MOUNTAIN	Between spring/ summer + summer/ autumn	G in cold/ C in hot	G autumn/ L other	C in hot/ L in cold	G autumn/ C summer/ L spring

Index

A

ama, 41–42, 48, 58, 134
Amaranth Kitchari with Cajun
   Veggies and Cranberry Pepper
   Chutney, 108–109
Apple Cranberry Chutney, 64
Apricot Cherry Sauce, Cinnamon
   Millet Porridge with, 103
astringent taste, 31–32
autumn, 36
Ayurveda
   Ayurvedic doctors, 137
   body-mind types, 17–26
   building actions, 42
   defined, 10
   definition of health, 13–14
   food-medicine, 30–35
   four steps to health, 10
   goals of, 11–13
   lightening actions, 42
   longevity goal, 12–13
   observation walk, 15
   principle of opposites, 14–15
   six stages of disease, 43–44
   spice-medicines, 35–37
   steps to cultivate health, 13
   traditional Ayurvedic cleansing,
      133–137

B

Banana-Berry Delight Sauce, Gingery
   Oatmeal Squares with, 84–85
beans
   Amaranth Kitchari with Cajun
      Veggies and Cranberry Pepper
      Chutney, 108–109
   Beans and Greens with Cashew
      Miso Tofu, 92–93
   Kitchari, 61
   mung beans, types of, 60
   Roasted Poblano Stuffed with
      Chickpeas and Spinach, 105
   Spring Secrets Vegetable Chili, 113
beets, 87
bellows breath, 97
bitter taste, 31–32
Black Rice and Cashew Porridge, 83

blood-letting, 134–135
body-mind types (doshas), 17–26
breathing practices, 75, 97, 117
Breeze type (vata)
   in balance, 23
   cleansing guidelines, 45
   color of imbalances, 43
   cycle of the day, 38–39
   grounding cleanse & diet, 69–93
   ideal foods, 32–33, 35
   nature, 19
   physical constitution, 19
   principle of movement, 25
   qualities, 18–19
   signs of imbalance, 24
   sleep needs, 39
   water needs, 49
burps, 54
Butter, Clarified (Ghee), 63

C

calming foods, 55
cardiovascular exercise, 97
chia seeds, 125
Chili, Spring Secrets Vegetable, 113
chutney
   Apple Cranberry Chutney, 64
   Coconut Cilantro Chutney, 64
   Cranberry Pepper Chutney,
      108–109
   Raisin Coconut Chutney, 64
cinnamon
   Cinnamon Millet Porridge with
      Apricot Cherry Sauce, 103
   Spiced Honey, 66
cleansing, 44–49. See also; dietary
   cleanse; digestive cleansing
   Ayurvedic vs. modern, 49
   Breeze type guidelines, 45
   categories of, 47–49
   contraindications for, 46
   evaluating imbalances for, 44
   Fire type guidelines, 46–47
   Mountain type guidelines, 45–46
   seasonal, 47
   when to cleanse, 44–45
Cleansing Table, 140–141
Coconut Cilantro Chutney, 64
coffee, note about, 122

Constitution Checklist
   filling out, 23
   questionnaire, 138
   using results to choose cleanse,
      140–141
cooling breath, 117
cooling cleanse, 46–47, 116–132
cornmeal
   Lighten Up Polenta with Squash
      Sauce, 112
   Savory Corn Grits with Spicy Kale,
      106
cranberries
   Apple Cranberry Chutney, 64
   Cranberry Pepper Chutney,
      108–109
cycle of the day, 37–39, 56–57
cycle of the seasons, 36–37

D

daily cleansing practices, 47
daily eating, 37–39, 56–57
dietary cleanse
   choosing right type, 57–58,
      140–141
   defined, 48
   examples of, 48
   for Breeze type, 77–79
   for Fire type, 118–120
   for Mountain type, 99–101
digestion
   improving, tips for, 100
   process of, 33
digestive cleansing
   defined, 48
   examples of, 48
   in last days of 31-day protocol, 58
   process of, 33
digestive fire
   balanced, 41–49
   in Fire types, 35
   imbalanced, 41–49
   influencing factors, 54
disease, six stages of, 43–44
drinks
   The Cool-Down "Iced" Tea, 121
   Elevate Me Tea, 104
   Indian Chocolate Spice, 81
   Turmeric "Latte," 122–123
dulling foods, 55, 56

E
elimination cleansing, 48–49
enemas, 135
exercise, 97, 118

F
fat, or adipose tissue, 42
Fire type (pitta)
    in balance, 26
    cleansing guidelines, 46–47
    color of imbalances, 43
    cooling cleanse & diet, 116–132
    cycle of the day, 37–38
    digestive fire, 35
    ideal foods, 34–35, 36
    intellectual abilities and ambitions, 22
    nature, 22
    physical constitution, 21, 22
    principle of temperature regulation and transformation, 25
    qualities, 21
    signs of imbalance, 26
    sleep needs, 39
    water needs, 49
food
    daily eating, 37–39
    food-medicine, 30–35
    mono diet, 45, 48, 58
    potency of, 30
    for predominant imbalance, 36–37
    seasonal eating, 36–37
fruit. *See also; specific fruits*
    Summer Sunrise Pudding, 125

G
ghee cleanse, 136–137
ginger
    Elevate Me Tea, 104
    Gingery Oatmeal Squares with Banana-Berry Delight Sauce, 84–85
    Lemon-Ginger-Honey Nectar, 67
    qualities of, 66
    Spiced Honey, 66
grounding cleanse, 45, 69–93
group cleansing, 48

H
health, defined, 13–14
herbalized oils, 71
honey
    Lemon-Ginger-Honey Nectar, 67
    Spiced Honey, 66

I
Imbalance Checklist, 26, 139, 140–141
immune system, 42

K
Kale, Spicy, Savory Corn Grits with, 106
Kitchari
    Amaranth Kitchari with Cajun Veggies and Cranberry Pepper Chutney, 108–109
    ingredients in, 60
    recipe for, 61
Konji and Porridge, Breakfast, 62

L
Lemon-Ginger-Honey Nectar, 67
lightening cleanse, 45–46, 95–114
lightening practices, 42, 48
longevity, 12–13
lymphatic system, 42

M
massage
    oil self-massage, 70–74, 117
    raw silk massage, 96–97
meal rituals, 56
meditation, 75
Millet Cinnamon Porridge with Apricot Cherry Sauce, 103
mindful eating, 54–56
mono diet, 45, 48, 58
morning routine, 57
Mountain type (kapha)
    in balance, 24
    cleansing guidelines, 45–46
    color of imbalances, 43
    cycle of the day, 37
    ideal foods, 33–34, 35–36
    lightening cleanse & diet, 95–114
    nature, 20–21
    physical constitution, 20
    principle of structure and stability, 25
    qualities, 20
    signs of imbalance, 24–25
    sleep needs, 39
    water needs, 49

N
naps, 67

O
Oatmeal Squares, Gingery, with Banana-Berry Delight Sauce, 84–85
oil
    herbalized oils, 71
    removing from cloth, 72
    self-massage, 70–74, 117
oleation, 47, 48, 135
onions, cooked vs. raw, 92
opposites, pairs of, 14–15

P
panchakarma
    with Ayurvedic professional, 137
    cleansing actions, 133–134
    elimination phases, 48–49
    first stage, 48, 134
    fourth stage, 136
    ghee cleanse, 136–137
    rejuvenation period, 136
    second stage, 134–135
    third stage, 135–136
peppermint, 104
peppers
    Cranberry Pepper Chutney, 108–109
    Roasted Poblano Stuffed with Chickpeas and Spinach, 105
Polenta, Lighten Up, with Squash Sauce, 112
porridge
    Black Rice and Cashew Porridge, 83
    Breakfast Porridge and Konji, 62
    Cinnamon Millet Porridge with Apricot Cherry Sauce, 103
portion size, 54

Pudding, Summer Sunrise, 125
pungent taste, 31–32
purgation with castor oil, 135

R
Raisin Coconut Chutney, 64
rejuvenation period, 136
rejuvenation practices, 49
rice
    basmati, 60
    Black Rice and Cashew Porridge, 83
    Breakfast Porridge and Konji, 62
    Kitchari, 61
right nostril breath, 97

S
salads
    Grilled Vegetables with Spring Bitters Salad and Sesame Garlic Dressing, 111
    Hijiki Rainbow Salad with Avocado Pumpkin-Seed Dressing, 130–131
salty taste, 31–32
seasonal cleansing, 47, 51
seasonal eating, 36–37
self-care practices
    for Breeze type, 69–77
    for Fire type, 116–118
    for Mountain type, 96–99
Slaw, Warm, 132
sleep, 39, 67
soups
    Golden Glow Soup, 87
    Sweet Green Goodness Soup with Cucumber Raita, 125–126
sour taste, 31–32
spice-medicines, 35–37
Spice Mixes, 65

Spinach and Chickpeas, Roasted Poblano Stuffed with, 105
spring, 36
Squash Sauce, Lighten Up Polenta with, 112
stevia, 34
stimulating foods, 55–56
sudation, 135
summer, 36
sweating, 97
sweet taste, 31–32

T
Tamarind Sauce, Belly-Warming Curried Roots with, 91
taste, and digestion, 33
tastes, six, 31–32
Tempeh and Stir-Fry Wrap, Tantalizing, 114
therapeutic vomiting, 135
31-day protocol, 53–59
    final cleansing days, 58
    modifying, 59
    staple recipes, 60–67
    transition time after, 59
    week 1, 54
    week 2, 54–56
    week 3, 56–57
    week 4, 57–58
tofu
    Beans and Greens with Cashew Miso Tofu, 92–93
    "Swami's Secret" Tofu Scramble, 124
tongue, reading the, 42–43
toxins, 42, 136
transition time, 59
turmeric
    Golden Glow Soup, 87
    Turmeric "Latte," 122–123

V
vegan or vegetarian diet, 48
vegetables. *See also specific vegetables*
    Amaranth Kitchari with Cajun Veggies and Cranberry Pepper Chutney, 108–109
    Beans and Greens with Cashew Miso Tofu, 92–93
    Belly-Warming Curried Roots with Tamarind Sauce, 91
    Green Beauty Sauté, 129
    Grilled Vegetables with Spring Bitters Salad and Sesame Garlic Dressing, 111
    Hijiki Rainbow Salad with Avocado Pumpkin-Seed Dressing, 130–131
    Spring Secrets Vegetable Chili, 113
    "Swami's Secret" Tofu Scramble, 124
    Sweet Green Goodness Soup with Cucumber Raita, 125–126
    Tantalizing Tempeh and Stir-Fry Wrap, 114
    Warm Slaw, 132
    Water-Sautéed Veggies, 88

W
water intake, 49
winter, 36

Y
yoga, bed, 58
yoga poses
    for Breeze type, 76–77
    for Fire type, 117–118
    for Mountain type, 98–99

CPSIA information can be obtained
at www.ICGtesting.com
Printed in the USA
BVHW060718221122
652431BV00002B/3